AF781180

REPRODUCTIVE HEALTH AND GENDER EQUALITY

To my parents and
my sister Guang-lan

Reproductive Health and Gender Equality

Method, Measurement, and Implications

GUANG-ZHEN WANG
University of Texas – Pan American, USA

ASHGATE

© Guang-zhen Wang 2010

All rights reserved. No part of this publication may be reproduced, stored in a retrieval system or transmitted in any form or by any means, electronic, mechanical, photocopying, recording or otherwise without the prior permission of the publisher.

Guang-zhen Wang has asserted her right under the Copyright, Designs and Patents Act, 1988, to be identified as the author of this work.

Published by
Ashgate Publishing Limited
Wey Court East
Union Road
Farnham
Surrey, GU9 7PT
England

Ashgate Publishing Company
Suite 420
101 Cherry Street
Burlington
VT 05401-4405
USA

www.ashgate.com

British Library Cataloguing in Publication Data
Wang, Guang-zhen.
Reproductive health and gender equality : method, measurement, and implications.
1. Reproductive health services--Developing countries--Research--Methodology.
2. Women--Health and hygiene--Developing countries--Research--Methodology.
3. Women's rights--Developing countries--Research--Metholodology. 4. Social status--Health aspects--Developing countries-- Research--Methodology. 5. Medical policy--Developing countries--Research--Methodology. 6. Health status indicators--Developing countries.
I. Title
613.9'082'091724-dc22

Library of Congress Cataloging-in-Publication Data
Wang, Guang-zhen.
Reproductive health and gender equality : method, measurement, and implications / by Guang-zhen Wang.
p. cm.
Includes bibliographical references and index.
ISBN 978-0-7546-4869-7 (hardback) -- ISBN 978-0-7546-9139-6 (ebook)
1. Reproductive health--Developing countries. 2. Women--Health and hygiene--Developing countries. 3. Women's rights--Developing countries. I. Title.
RA564.85.W357 2010
362.196'650091724--dc22

2010020880

ISBN 9780754648697 (hbk)
ISBN 9780754691396 (ebk)

Mixed Sources
Product group from well-managed forests and other controlled sources
www.fsc.org Cert no. SGS-COC-2482
© 1996 Forest Stewardship Council

Printed and bound in Great Britain by
TJ International Ltd, Padstow, Cornwall

Contents

List of Figures — *vii*
List of Tables — *ix*
Acronyms and Abbreviations — *xi*
Preface — *xv*
Acknowledgements — *xvii*

1 Overview — **1**
1.1 Introduction — 1
1.2 What is Women's Reproductive Health? — 5
1.3 Theoretical Perspectives — 7

2 Theoretical Explanations of the Proposed Model — **19**
2.1 Women's Human Rights and Reproductive Health — 19
2.2 Gender Equality and Women's Reproductive Health — 29
2.3 Maternal-Child Health Care and Women's Reproductive Health — 34
2.4 Economic Development and Gender Equality — 35
2.5 Political Development and Gender Equality — 37
2.6 Economic Development and Women's Human Rights — 38
2.7 Political Development and Women's Human Rights — 38
2.8 Economic Development and Maternal-Child Care — 39
2.9 Political Development and Maternal-Child Care — 39

3 Measurement of the Variables — **41**
3.1 Indicators and Scales of Women's Reproductive Health — 41
3.2 Indicators of Exogenous Variables — 58
3.3 Data Sources — 66

4 Findings and Analysis — **69**
4.1 Descriptive Statistics — 69
4.2 Measurement Model — 81
4.3 Structural Model — 83
4.4 Alternative Model — 86

5 Regional Variations — **91**
5.1 Regional Variations in Women's Reproductive Health Indicators — 92
5.2 Cluster Analysis — 94

5.3 OLS Estimates of Regional Variations 98
5.4 The sub-Saharan Africa Dilemma 100

6 Discussion and Implications 107
6.1 Enhancing Gender Equality Approach to Women's Reproductive Health 107
6.2 Engendering Social Policies in Light of Women's Reproductive Health 111
6.3 Limitations of the Study 116
6.4 Summary 118

Appendix A Millennium Development Goals (MDGs), Targets, and Indicators 121
Appendix B Declaration of the Rights of Man and the Citizen, 26 August 1789 127
Appendix C Chronology of International Conferences on Gender Equality, Women's Rights, and Women's Reproductive Health 129
Appendix D Women's Human Rights and Reproductive Rights 135
Appendix E Developing Countries in Regional Aggregates 141
Appendix F Reproductive Health among Refugees and Internally Displaced Persons List of Selected Websites 143
Appendix G Global Gag Rule Timeline 145
Appendix H President Obama's Memorandum (January 23, 2009) 159
Appendix I List of Selected Non-governmental Organizations (NGOs) Women's Reproductive Health and Reproductive Rights 161
Appendix J Countries in Major World Aggregates 169
Appendix K Countries or Areas in Income Aggregates 171

Bibliography *173*
Index *199*

List of Figures

2.1	Proposed Model	40
4.1	The Findings of the Structural Model	86
4.2	Alternative Model	88
4.3	Q-Plot Comparison: Structural Model and Alternative Model	89
5.1	Comparison of Regional Variations	95

List of Tables

3.1	WHO, UNICEF, and UNFPA: List of Reproductive Health Indicators 1993–1996	43
3.2	Hierarchy of Reproductive Health Indicators	49
3.3	CDC Reproductive Health Indicators	51
3.4	Chronology of Reproductive Health Indicators	53
3.5	Variables and Data Sources	68
4.1	Descriptive Statistics	70
4.2	Analysis of the Variables	73
4.3	Measurement Model Parameters	82
4.4	Structural Model, LISREL Estimates	83
4.5	Alternative Structural Model, LISREL Estimates	87
5.1	Regional Variations: Maternal Mortality (per 100,000 live births)	92
5.2	Regional Variations: Infant Mortality (per 1,000 live births)	93
5.3	Regional Variations: Percentage Infants with Low Birth Weight (less than 2,500 grams)	94
5.4	Cluster Analysis: Women's Reproductive Health	96
5.5	Selected Social and Economic Characteristics of the Least Developed Countries	97
5.6	OLS Estimates of the Effects of Regional Variables on Women's Reproductive Health	98

Acronyms and Abbreviations

ACRJ	Asian Communities for Reproductive Justice
AGFI	adjusted goodness of fit
AGI	Alan Guttmacher Institute
AGIL	Adaptation, Goal attainment, Integration, Latency
AI	Amnesty International
AIDS	acquired immunodeficiency syndrome
ANC	antenatal care
ARHNe	Adolescent Reproductive Health Network
AWDF	African Women's Development Fund
CAFS	Center for African Family Studies
CAPRISA	Centre for the AIDS Program of Research in South Africa
CAPS	Center for AIDS Prevention Studies
CDC	Centers for Disease Control and Prevention
CEDAW	Convention on the Elimination of All Forms of Discrimination against Women
CEDPA	Center for Development and Population Activities
CFA	confirmatory factor analysis
CHANGE	Center for Health and Gender Equity
CIRI	(The) Cingranelli-Richards Human Rights Dataset
CPR	contraceptive prevalence rate
CRC	Convention on the Rights of the Child
CRLP	Center for Reproductive Law and Policy
CRR	Center for Reproductive Rights
CRWH	Coalition for Research in Women's Health
CSA	Center for the Study of AIDS in South Africa
CSDH	Commission on Social Determinants of Health
CSW	Commission on the Status of Women
DAC	(OECD's) Development Assistance Committee
DAWN	Development Alternatives with Women for a New Era
DOW	Doctors of the World
DRH	(CDC's) Division of Reproductive Health
ECOD	economic development
ECOSOC	United Nations Economic and Social Council
EOC	essential obstetric care
ESCAP	United Nations Economic and Social Commission for Asia and the Pacific
EU	European Union

FAO	Food and Agriculture Organization
FGM	female genital mutilation
FHI	Family Health International
FIGO	International Federation of Gynecology and Obstetrics
GDI	Gender Development Index
GDP	gross domestic product
GEI	Gender Equality Index
GEM	Gender Empowerment Measure
GEND	gender equality
GESDI	Gross Environment Sustainable Development Index
GFATM	Global Fund to Fight AIDS, Tuberculosis, and Malaria
GFI	goodness of fit
GKN	Globalization Knowledge Network
GNP	Gross National Product
GPI	Genuine Progress Indicator
GRHF	Global Reproductive Health Forum, Harvard University
GSDP	Gross Sustainable Development Product
HAIN	Health Action Information Network
HCHR	Office of the High Commissioner for Human Rights
HDI	Human Development Index
HDN	Health and Development Networks
HDPDS	Harvard Center for Population and Development Studies
HIPCs	(External Debt Management in) Heavily Indebted Poor Countries
HIV	human immunodeficiency virus
IAAH	International Association for Adolescent Health
IAWG	Inter-agency Working Group on Refugee Reproductive Health
IBCR	International Bureau for Children's Rights
ICAP	International Center for AIDS Care and Treatment Programs
ICOMP	International Council on Management of Population Programmes
ICPD	International Conference on Population and Development
ICRH	International Center for Reproductive Health
ICW	International Council of Women
IDP	internally displaced people
IDPs	internally displaced persons
IFFA	International Federation of Fertility Societies
IFRC	Federation for International Cooperation of Health Services and Systems Research Centers
IHG	international health governance
IHP	International Health Partnership
ILO	International Labor Organization
IMF	International Monetary Fund
IOWD	International Organization for Women and Development
IPPF	International Planned Parenthood Federation
IPU	Inter-Parliamentary Union

IRC	International Rescue Committee
ITU	International Telecommunication Fund
IUSTI	International Union against Sexually Transmitted Infections
IWHC	International Women's Health Coalition
LACWHN	Latin American and Caribbean Women's Health Network
LDCs	least developed countries
MCHC	maternal-child care
MDGs	Millennium Development Goals
MDRI	Multilateral Debt Relief Initiative
MISP	Minimum Initial Service Package
MMR	maternal mortality rate
ODA	Official Development Assistance
ODP	Ocean Drilling Programme
OECD	Official Economic Co-operation and Development
OLS	Ordinary Least Square models
PAI	Population Action International
PNMR	perinatal mortality rate
POLD	political development
POPIN	United Nations Population Information Network
PPFA	Planned Parenthood Federation of America
PRB	Population Reference Bureau
PRC	Population Resources Center
PSI	Population Services International
RHRC	Reproductive Health for Refugees Consortium
RMSR	root mean square residual
SARA	Support for Analysis and Research in Africa
SDHE	social determinants for health equity
SDPs	service delivery points
SEM	structural equation modeling
SMC	squared multiple correlation
STDs	sexually transmitted diseases
TBAs	trained health personnel
TFR	total fertility rate
UN	United Nations
UNAIDS	United Nations Joint Programme on HIV/AIDS (The Joint United Nations Programme on HIV/AIDS)
UNDESA	United Nations Department of Economic and Social Affairs
UNDP	United Nations Development Programme
UNEP	United Nations Environment Programme
UNESA	United Nations Economic and Social Affairs
UNESCO	United Nations Educational, Scientific, and Cultural Organization
UNFPA	United Nations Fund for Population Activities
UNGASS	United Nations General Assembly Special Session
UNHCR	United Nations High Commissioner for Refugees

UNHCHR	Office of the High Commissioner for Human Rights
UNICEF	United Nations Children's Fund
UNIFEM	United Nations Development Fund for Women
USAID	United States Agency for International Development
WCRWC	Women's Commission for Refugee Women and Children
WFPHA	World Federation of Public Health Association
WGNRR	Women's Global Network for Reproductive Rights
WHO	World Health Organization
WHOSIS	World Health Organization – Statistical Information System
WOMR	women's human rights
WORH	women's reproductive health
WRA	women of reproductive age

Preface

This book is neither about the behavioral correlates of women's reproductive health nor about the clinical account on safe motherhood or child survival. The book goes beyond the capacity of many of the previous publications on this topic by emphasizing three components. First, it provides a conceptual and operational framework of women's reproductive health and the other variables used in this study, including gender equality, women's human rights, and political and economic development. Second, the analyses are limited to country-level data. Inferences are drawn from the data obtained from 137 developing countries (or areas). Third, this book features an empirical study by testing the impact of gender equality, women's human rights, and maternal-child care on women's reproductive health within the context of economic and political development and explores the theoretical and social policy implications based on the findings from the proposed model. This approach owes its origin to the study of women's reproductive rights and reproductive health pioneered by Betsy Hartmann (1987), Rebecca J. Cook (1993), Ruth Dixon-Mueller (1993), Sonia Correa and Rosalind Petchesky (1994), Gita Sen (1994), and Susan McDaniel (1996).

Since the 1994 International Conference on Population and Development (ICPD), the rhetoric about the linkages between gender equality and women's reproductive health has been more than ever the focal point among policy makers and advocates in the international community. For example, the report by the World Health Organization (WHO 2004) acknowledged that the lack of socioeconomic opportunities for women is the underlying cause of women's reproductive health problems. The United Nations Fund for Population Activities (UNFPA 2005), in its *State of World Population* report associated women's reproductive health with social justice and gender equality.

In spite of the growing concerns with women's reproductive health especially in developing countries, social science research on reproductive health, as Matthews, Ribar, and Wilhelm (1997), Parker (2001, 2002), and Östlin (2004) have recognized, is mostly descriptive and focuses on behavioral correlates among individuals. Empirical research on the relationship between gender-based power relations and sexual and reproductive health outcomes is scarce (Blanc 2001, Commission on Social Determinants of Health – CSDH 2008). Scientific inquiries are, to a large extent, inadequate in looking into the potential explanations for maternal and infant health that are mainly rooted in women's social, economic, and political histories (Bennett 1997, Östlin, Schrecker, and Sadana 2009). In addition, methodological issues in terms of the conceptualization and the construction of operational indicators to measure women's reproductive health and gender equality related variables have not been adequately addressed (Sadana 2002, Wang 2007).

Presser (1997) and Hanefeld, Spicer, Brugha, and Walt (2007) pointed out that research attempt that more broadly relates gender relations to demographic behavior in an international context and incorporates development issues at large has emerged only recently and that this type of research is limited in scope and fragmented. Östlin, Schrecker, and Sadana (2009) urged social scientists to adopt research focusing on how global contexts affect health inequalities especially women's reproductive health in developing countries.

This book grew out of years of my research on women's reproductive rights and reproductive health. It is an attempt to add to the academic literature for an empirical study of women's reproductive health in developing countries using a gender equality approach.

Guang-zhen Wang

Acknowledgements

I sincerely acknowledge the anonymous reviewers for their extensive commentaries on the prospectus and the chapters of the book. Special thanks are due to my husband, Dr Lucian Spataro whose complete understanding was extremely important for me to concentrate on this work.

The editors at Ashgate Publishing, especially Mary Savigar, Carolyn Court, Neil Jordan and Nikki Selmes have provided efficient and professional attention to the publication of the book, for which I am very grateful.

Chapter 1
Overview

This chapter provides an overview of women's reproductive health in developing countries (or areas). It is divided into two sections. The first section discusses the propensities in current research on women's reproductive health and the organization of the book. The second section focuses on the discussions of the three major perspectives that have evolved during the last few decades with regard to women's reproductive health: the neo-Malthusian thought and the demographic perspective, the public health perspectives, and the gender equality approach.

1.1 Introduction

Women's reproductive health is a very sensitive issue and it tends to be tangled up with the wide spectrum of social justice, such as women's social, economic, and political status; human rights; population policies; and cultural integrity (Cook 1995, Hellsten 2000, McDaniel 2002, Wickrama and Lorenz 2002, Keleher and Franklin 2008). The World Health Organization (WHO) declared in its 2008 report that social justice is a matter of life and death and that inequality in the social, political, and economic conditions determines the risk of illnesses and women's health including their reproductive health. Reproductive health is also critical to the well-being of women and children. According to the World Bank (2008) and the United Nations Fund for Population Activities (UNFPA 2008), about 200 million women, mostly in developing countries, suffer from pregnancy and childbirth related life-threatening complications and disabilities. As a result, an estimated 250 million years of productive life are lost every year. Pregnancy and childbirth are the leading cause of death and disability for women of reproductive age in developing countries (World Bank 2008). However, about a couple of decades ago, much of the world's attention centered on how to slow down the high population growth rates in most of the developing countries (Wang and Pillai 2001).

Beginning in the mid-1990s, a number of international conferences were held and women's reproductive rights and reproductive health issues particularly in developing countries became the focal agenda. The 1994 United Nations International Conference on Population and Development (ICPD), known as the Cairo Conference, adopted the Programme of Action. It endorsed a new strategy that links the demographic goals of reducing population size to the improvement of infant, child, and maternal mortality and women's reproductive health conditions. The ICPD's Programme of Action drew up an ambitious plan to make reproductive health in developing countries a major international priority. The

1995 Fourth World Conference on Women (Beijing Conference) reaffirmed the goals and objectives of the 1994 Cairo Conference. In June 2000, representatives from 180 countries met at the United Nations Headquarters in New York City for the five-year review of the implementation of the Programme of Action and the Beijing Platform of Action. The review confirmed the centrality of gender equality, reproductive rights, and sustainable development in advancing women's reproductive health worldwide. Five years later in 2005, world leaders gathered again at the United Nations Headquarters for the World Summit. The World Summit, the largest gathering in history, reiterated the international commitment to the Millennium Development Goals (MDGs) and the need to keep reproductive health, gender equality, and economic development at the top of the world development agenda.[1] The state leaders at the World Summit recognized that HIV/AIDS and other infectious and reproductive health problems and diseases had posed severe risks to the achievement of world development goals and the Summit called for a full implementation of the MDGs to ensure reproductive health services, improve maternal health, and reduce infant and child mortality. The World Health Organization (WHO 2006), meanwhile, identified three reproductive health-related MDGs: reduce child mortality, improve maternal health, and combat HIV/AIDS as the most important challenges facing the world health system today.

In spite of the recent changes in rhetoric from an emphasis on demographic goals of reducing population size in developing countries to the recognition of promoting women's reproductive health through sustainable development and the enhancement of gender equality, progress has been very slow (Ashford 2001, Woodward and Simms 2006, World Health Organization 2009). Maternal and infant mortality is still among the worst performing health indicator in resource-poor countries and regions (Say, Souza, and Patterson 2009), and it has barely changed since 1990 (World Health Organization 2009). About 95 percent of the maternal deaths and 90 percent of the new-born deaths have occurred in developing countries (United Nations Children's Fund 2009), and most of these deaths are preventable (Save the Children Fund 2006). In addition, more than one quarter of all adult women living in developing countries currently suffer from short or long term illnesses and injuries related to pregnancy and childbirths (United Nations Children's Fund 2009).

1 The United Nations member states have pledged to meet the Millennium Development Goals (MDGs) by 2015. There are eight Millennium Development Goals (United Nations Development Pprogram 2006, World Bank 2008): (1) Eradicate extreme poverty and hunger; (2) Achieve universal primary education; (3) Promote gender equality and empower women; (4) Reduce child mortality; (5) Improve maternal health; (6) Combat HIV/AIDS, malaria and other diseases; (7) Ensure environmental sustainability; and (8) Develop global partnership for development (Appendix A. Millennium Development Goals, Targets, and Indicators).

As Merali (2000) and Östlin (2004) stated, on a global scale, especially in developing countries, women's reproductive health and reproductive rights have been denied, ignored, and violated. Rosenfield and Schwartz (2005) further claimed that the issue of women's reproductive health ranks at the bottom of the international community's list of priorities. The statistics recounted in *The State of World Population* (United Nations Fund for Population Activities 2009) painted a heartrending picture of the reproductive lives of hundreds of thousands of women living in developing countries. Here are some of the examples: more than 585,000 women die each year in developing countries, about 1,600 deaths each day, for reasons related to pregnancy and childbirth and at rates 200 times higher than those in industrialized countries. There are no trained birth attendants available to assist at 60 million births each year, and fewer than 30 percent of the mothers in developing countries as a whole receive postpartum care, compared with an average of 90 percent in industrialized countries. Almost half of the 175 million pregnancies that occur each year in developing countries are unwanted or ill-timed, and the number is probably higher, given the often insufficient data on adolescent female pregnancies. Ilona Kickbusch (2004) noted the huge gap in infant and maternal deaths between developed and developing countries: infant mortality rate is 5.1 per 1,000 live births in Canada and 97.1 in Haiti, under five mortality rate is 16.5 times greater in Haiti than that in Canada, and maternal mortality rate is 35 times higher in Latin America and the Caribbean than that in North America. According to the 2009 United Nations Children's Fund report (UNICEF 2009), for a woman in a least developed country, the average lifetime risk of dying from complications related to pregnancy and childbirth is more than 300 times greater than that for a woman living in an industrialized country. No other mortality rate is so unequal.

In spite of all of that, empirical research on reproductive health and gender equality is inadequate and still remains "a neglected area" (Lane 1994, Wang and Pillai 2001, Commission on Social Determinants of Health, World Health organization 2008). As Presser (1997) and Nelson (2000) reminded us, while the ICPD's Program of Action has advocated the empowerment of women and gender equality, we are still lacking sufficient scientific knowledge about how and to what extent gender equality and women's human rights are related to the demographic processes in the area of women's reproductive health. Östlin (2004) further argued that understanding the social dimension of women's health, particularly reproductive health, generally falls outside the frame of reference and that "even the current focus of most non-biomedical health research is predominantly on individual risk factors; and the social context that frames the distribution and modifies the effect of these risk factors is often neglected." (p. 8).

In reviewing current research on women's reproductive health, I have found the following propensities. First, research on women's reproductive health is mostly descriptive and focuses on the behavioral correlates among individuals (Matthews, Ribar, and Wilhelm 1997, Parker 2001, 2002). Most literature on women's reproductive health is either clinical or exclusively deals with women's health problems (Qadeer 1998, Sen, George, and Östlin 2002). Academic research on the theoretical and empirical linkages between reproductive health and social, economic and political factors has been minimal and inadequate (Bird and Bauman 1995, Stivens 2000, Wittrock 2000, Marks 2001a, 2001b, Östlin, Schrecker, and Sadana 2009). As Presser (1997) and Hanefeld, Spicer, Brugha, and Walt (2007) pointed out, one of the deficiencies of reproductive health research to date is the small number of rigorous quantitative models that specify the links between gender-based power relations and sexual and reproductive health outcomes. In response to the lack of such research endeavor, the World Health Organization (WHO) Task Force on Research Priorities (2005) called for health research to improve the understanding of the effects of social context on health outcome for populations and to "examine the links between proximal and structural determinants of ill-health and study the institutions and processes leading to health inequalities." (p. 949). In 2008, the Commission on Social Determinants of Health (CSDH) of the World Health Organization (WHO) issued its final report, identifying actions on the understanding of the social determinants of health as one of its three overarching tasks. The World Health Assembly's 2009 resolution called for urgent research agenda to address the social determinants and social gradients of health and health inequalities.

Second, methodological issues related to the conceptualization and the constructions of operational indicators to measure women's reproductive health, gender equality, and women's human rights have not been adequately addressed (Sadana 2002, Wang 2007). Recent indicator validation studies have shown a lack of the conceptual and operational meanings of the key concepts in reproductive health research (Jacobson 2000, Sadana 2002). Sen, George, and Östlin (2002) further argued for a quantitative research methodology in health and human rights research with variables properly defined and adequately measured. Sadana (2002) suggested two challenges in developing and testing practical indicators of reproductive health, one of the challenges is "how a conceptual definition of reproductive health – focusing on human condition – may serve as a basis for operational indicators." (pp. 407–408). The first internationally recognized definition of reproductive health that incorporated the World Health Organization's (WHO 1948) constitutional designation of health in general was adopted at the 1994 International Conference on Population and Development (ICPD 1994). Although progress has been made since then in terms of the data availability pertaining to reproductive health and reproductive rights at the national and international levels, the conceptual definitions of reproductive health and other relevant variables that are meaningful across populations have been highly controversial within the research community, and in addition, there is still certain obscurity in terms of the validations of the measurement.

This book serves three purposes. First, the book attempts to provide a conceptual and operational framework of women's reproductive health and the other variables used in this study. Conceptual framework and the measurement of women's reproductive health, gender equality, women's rights, maternal-child care, economic and political development are presented in Chapter 2 and Chapter 3.

Second, the analyses are limited to country-level data. Inferences are drawn from data obtained from 137 developing countries (or areas).[2] Greenhalgh (1990) and Hanefeld, Spicer, Brugha, and Walt (2007) have called for research operating at regional, national, and global levels. Östlin, Schrecker, and Sadana (2009), further, urged social scientists to adopt research focusing on how global contexts affect health inequalities especially women's reproductive health in developing countries. Third, the book attempts to provide an empirical study by testing the impact of gender equality, women's rights, and maternal-child care on women's reproductive health within the context of economic and political development and explores the theoretical and social policy implications based on the findings from the proposed model. Blanc (2001) reiterated the need for quantitative research in the field, arguing that "In many studies, an observed outcome is assumed to be the result of a gender-based power dynamic that is speculated on or buttressed with qualitative information. Power relations themselves are rarely measured (in qualitative studies); thus if a desirable outcome occurs, attributing it to a change in power relations is often impossible." (Blanc 2001: 206).

The book is divided into six chapters and organized in the following way. Chapter 1 provides an overview of women's reproductive health. This chapter includes three sections: (1) Introduction, (2) What is Women's Reproductive Health? and (3) Theoretical Perspectives. Chapter 2 is devoted to the discussion of the conceptual framework of the proposed model and the explanations of women's reproductive health in relation to the exogenous dimensions. Chapter 3 discusses the measurement of the variables used in this study. Chapter 4 focuses on the statistical analyses of the proposed model. The proposed model is tested using structural equation analysis. Chapter 5 explores variations in women's reproductive health in sub-Saharan Africa, Arab States, East Asia/Pacific, South Asia, Latin American/Caribbean, and Southern Europe/Central Asia. Using OLS (ordinary least square models) and cluster analysis, this chapter examines the effect of the region variables on women's reproductive health. Chapter 6 discusses theoretical and social policy implications and limitations of the study based on the findings from the 137 developing countries. A brief summary is presented at the end of the chapter.

1.2 What is Women's Reproductive Health?

The term reproductive health is not new to medical professionals. The biomedical view of health has dominated the science literature for a very long time and was

2 The United Nations Development Programme (UNDP 2008) in its *Human Development Report 2007-2008* (p. 376) identified 137 developing countries. Available at: http://hdr.undp.org/en/media/HDR_20072008_EN_complete.pdf. Data from developing countries provide for sufficient variations of hypothesized independent and dependent dimensions.

only called into question in the last decades. The biologically oriented model sees health as a condition which remains after illnesses and dysfunctions are factored out. Health professionals and medicine have conscientiously looked for physiological and psychiatric causes of ill health (Cook 1995, Sadik 2000, Sen, Heorge, and Östlin 2002). Reproductive health or health in general is often associated with a physiological malfunction that results in an actual or potential reduction in the physical and reproduction-related activities and/or a reduced life span.

The 1994 International Conference on Population and Development (ICPD 1994) is considered to be the turning point in redefining reproductive health. Representatives from 1,254 non-governmental organizations all over the world produced a 20-year plan of action (Programme of Action) commending a new strategy of universal access to reproductive health care; reducing infant, child, and maternal deaths; better education, especially for girls; equality between men and women; and sustainable development. All of the representatives at the Conference agreed that women's reproductive health is important in its own right and that population control objectives should be integrated into the broader social development goals and women's reproductive health needs (Feitshans 1998, Ashford 2001). Women's reproductive health issues have since attained higher international visibility and renewed political commitment, a sharp contrast to the stance of the earlier decades when much of the world's attention focused on slowing down the population growth rates especially in Asia and sub-Saharan Africa. As identified in the ICPD's Programme of Action, reproductive health was defined as:

> a state of complete physical, mental and social well-being and not merely the absence of disease or infirmity, in all matters relating to the reproductive system and to its functions and processes. Reproductive health therefore implies that people are able to have a satisfying and safe sex life and that they have the capability to reproduce and the freedom to decide if, when and how often to do so. Implicit in this last condition are the rights of men and women to be informed and to have access to safe, effective, affordable and acceptable methods of family planning of their choice, as well as other methods of their choice for regulation of fertility which are not against the law, and the right of access to appropriate health-care services that will enable women to go safely through pregnancy and childbirth and provide couples with the best chance of having a healthy infant. (Programme of Action, paragraph 7.2)

In this first internationally agreed-upon definition of reproductive health, three interconnected implications are apparent. First, women's reproductive health goes far beyond reproduction and population control. It is important in and of itself. Women's reproductive health must be a global priority. Second, women's reproductive health is a basic human right to be fulfilled by all governments. And third, women's reproductive health seeks to address the underlying causes of gender equality and sustainable development (Sadik 2000, Rosenfield and Schwartz 2005).

1.3 Theoretical Perspectives

Over the past decades, three major distinctive perspectives have evolved with regard to women's reproductive health. These perspectives have spawned additional versions of women's reproductive health. The demographic perspective, which is grounded in neo-Malthusian thought, mostly focuses on contraceptive effectiveness and the aggregate goals of reducing population size particularly in developing countries with very little concern about women's reproductive health. The traditional public health model is mostly concerned with identifying patterns of diseases and disorders among certain groups of people and improving the health of a population by preventive medicine, health education, and the monitoring of environmental hazards. The gender equality approach views women's reproductive health in line with gender relations in the society. This section provides a brief review of the three major perspectives.

I. Neo-Malthusian Thought and the Demographic Perspective

The neo-Malthusian claim rests heavily on Thomas Malthus' *An Essay on the Principle of Population* (1789), in which Malthus argued that population increases exponentially and that subsistence increases arithmetically. As a consequence, human beings will live at a bare subsistence level. Malthus' theory is fundamentally based on the relationship between population and food production. As early as the1880s, neo-Malthusians opened up clinics to pass on messages of birth control. The Madras neo-Malthusian League in India (founded in 1882), for instance, blamed the poor for their own fate, claiming that the impoverishment of the lower class is a result of population increase among them and that a check on population growth through birth control would help improve the standard of living of the poor.

By the end of the 1950s, the number of the countries that were perceived to have "population problems" had expanded from countries in Asia to nearly all of the third world countries (Hodgson and Watkins 1997). How to slow down rapid population growth rates in low-income countries thus became a major concern of the whole world, while very little attention was given to women's reproductive health and their reproductive rights. Demographic researchers, such as Notestein (1950), Moore (1956), Osborn (1960), and Coale (1973) developed various models that quantify the economic costs of continued population growth. Greissimer (1954), in his booklet, warned that population growth has threatened to create an explosion as disruptive and dangerous as an atomic explosion. The issue of population growth, more specifically, overpopulation became the focal point of academic research and government policies during that time. China's one-child-per-couple policy that officially started in 1979 was among those policies and practices that reflect the neo-Malthusian belief that rapid and uncontrolled population growth is detrimental to the environment and societal development and will present a potentially insurmountable obstacle to social and economic development and the enjoyment of human rights.

In 1968, two influential neo-Malthusian works were published: one was Paul Ehrlich's *Population Bomb*, and the other, Garrett Hardin's *Tragedy of the Commons*. They both depicted a catastrophic picture as a result of the rapid increase in population size. Ehrlich (1968) envisioned an imminent global tragedy in which hundreds of millions of people will starve to death if the number of people on earth keeps going up. Ehrlich and Ehrlich (1972) further proposed laws that would make the act of bearing a third child illegal and require an abortion to terminate all such pregnancies. Hardin's (1968) essay introduced a hypothetical pasture as an analogy for "commons." To maximize personal gains, local herders increase their herd size, and consequently, the cattle die due to overgrazing and degradation of the pasture. Here's how Hardin (1968) described the tragedy of the commons.

> Picture a pasture open to all. It is to be expected that each herdsman will try to keep as many cattle as possible on the commons. Such an arrangement may work reasonably satisfactorily for centuries because tribal wars, poaching, and disease keep the numbers of both man and beast well below the carrying capacity of the land. Finally, however, comes the day of reckoning, that is the day when long-desired goal of social stability becomes a reality. At this point, the inherent logic of the commons remorselessly generates tragedy. (Hardin 1968: 1244)

The neo-Malthusian effort gained momentum in the 1970s, imposing substantial influence on public opinions and attracting political and economic resources. The original agenda of the World Population Conference at Bucharest in 1974 reflected the interest of neo-Malthusians to reduce population growth rates. Population control programs in developing countries were thus funded by the United States Agency for International Development (USAID), the World Bank, and other family planning and non-governmental organizations (NGOs).

The 1990s saw an explosion of the scholarship that was devoted to the study of population in relation to the environment, and human security (Schuwarts, Deligiannis, and Homer-Dixon 2000). Some of these scholarly works reflected the neo-Malthusian perspective. For example, Freeman and Isaacs (1993) suggested that "The grim scenarios of global devastation are beginning to fill the air." (p.21). Homer-Dixon (1991, 2000), in the discussion on the ingenuity gap, argued that we are caught between a soaring requirement for ingenuity and an increasingly uncertain supply due to the substantial increase in the number of people. As the ingenuity gap widens, political and violent upheavals will occur, which will adversely affect the economy and the well-being of the people. Homer-Dixon (2000) claimed that developing countries are likely to be affected sooner and more severely by population growth and environmental changes than industrial countries are because they lack political, social, financial, and intellectual resources. Another study by the United Nations Joint Programme on HIV/AIDS (UNAIDS 2006) found that the degradation of natural resources as a result of overpopulation is linked to higher mortality rates, particularly among women and children.

A number of scholars have recently questioned the validity of the neo-Malthusian theory. One of the criticisms is that the neo-Malthusian perspective is largely simplistic and ahistorical; and it ignored the political and economic causes of poverty, environmental degradation, and conflict. Richard Matthew (2000), for example, used Pakistan's North and West Provinces as a case study, arguing that the relationship between population growth and environmental conflict is complex and that environmental stress may either escalate conflict or reduce tensions and help resolve conflict. The neo-Malthusian thought and family planning programs especially in some developing countries have spawned two major concerns: one is concerned with the violation of human rights, in particular women's reproductive rights, and the other, with a possible increase in reproductive health risks.

II. Public Health Perspectives

The public health discipline emerged in Western Europe in the 18th century, around the same time as the European Enlightenment. Unlike clinical and medical practice, the classical public health field focuses on patterns of health and disease distributions as well as socioeconomic determinants of disease frequencies in populations. Epidemiology is a major tool that public health professionals draw on to study patterns of health and diseases. According to epidemiological transition theory, changes in the patterns of diseases take place in three stages. The first stage, also the longest stage, encompasses most human history. This stage is characterized by high general, infant, and maternal mortality rates; and most of these deaths can be traced to infectious diseases. The second stage is called receding pandemic. This stage sees a decrease in the prevalence of the diseases associated with those during the first stage. In Europe and North America, this shift occurred during the period between the middle of the 19th and the 20th centuries. The third stage in which industrialized nations have now found themselves is characterized by a high rate of degenerative and human-induced diseases such as cancer.

Explanations of epidemiological transition take into consideration economic and technological advancement and social structural changes. During the pre-agricultural era, humans were exposed to a large number of physical hazards and uncertainties about their sources and supplies of food due to the mode of sustenance. Life expectancy was very short and infant and maternal mortality rates were very high. With the advent of agriculture and the increase in population density, human populations became less nomadic and more complex and hierarchical forms of social organizations were created to control the production and the distribution of agricultural produce. As a result, the old social units based on primary and kin relationships were subordinated to the state and other large-scale institutions. More recently, a number of public health professionals sought to locate patterns of morbidity and mortality within the broad socioeconomic context. Thomas McKeown (1991), for example, has identified an array of social and economic determinants of health, including economic growth and social change, improved nutrition, and greater social and economic equality.

In the public health community, there are mainly two arguments regarding health and human rights. The first is what John Rawls (1921–2004) called "justice as fairness." According to Rawls (1971), there are two basic principles to attain justice or fairness. First, each person should get an equal guarantee to as many different liberties and as much of those liberties as can be guaranteed to everyone else at the same time. Second, inequalities in society are okay only if they are arranged in such a way that the inequalities actually help out the least fortunate persons in society; and only if the inequalities are connected to positions or offices or jobs in society that everyone has an equal opportunity to attain. An alternative argument implies that health is not a prerequisite for, but the consequence of individual choice. In Amartya Sen's (1973) terminology, the aim of health is to maximize the set of capacities available to individuals; and the level of functioning each person achieves is then their choice. Both arguments have been criticized for ignoring the social structural forces that directly affect human life and health outcomes.

In recent years, social scientists and feminist thinkers have raised a number of concerns about the ethical issues in public health practices. Marc Roberts and Michael Reich (2002) identified three serious ethical dilemmas facing the public health field. The first dilemma concerns whether public health policy decisions can be made on the basis of the calculation of their effect on the sum total of people's well-being (utilitarianism). The second dilemma deals with the controversy of whether health is a prerequisite for choice, or health is a consequence of choice, and how health rights relate to human rights. The third ethical dilemma sees to the subject of morality. Roberts and Reich (2002) further raised the question of whether there is a single true form of a good society and its associated virtues or whether each community defines its own virtues. One frequently asked question would be: Can female genital mutilation be justified by the so-called cultural respect?

III. Gender Equality Approach

The gender equality approach has offered a new way to understand and analyze the demographic processes of mortality and fertility (Basu 2000). The shift from a demographic goal-oriented practice to an approach that focuses on gender equality as an explanatory variable in analyzing women's reproductive health emerged in the recent decade. A number of social and political phenomena have played a catalytic role in the emergence and current visibility of the gender equality approach. The second wave feminist movement and the international women's health and women's rights movement during the late 1960s and 1970s are among the most influential forces.

The second wave feminist movement sparked by the civil rights movement and Betty Friedan's (1963) book *The Feminine Mystique* had considerable impact on the ideological shift from the demographic perspective to the gender equality approach. The second wave feminist movement, as a political actor, was mainly concerned with social justice and women's human rights, including women's reproductive rights and their right to choose. Early in the 1970s, Bonnie Mass (1972) strongly criticized the neo-Malthusian thought, claiming that demographic goals and birth controls are simply a part of a strategy to maintain Western hegemony by controlling the wombs of the third world women. Linda Gordon (1974) portrayed neo-Malthusians as eugenicists who strive to preserve "the hegemony of the most able of the old Yankees" by limiting the numbers and the influence of the world's nonwhite populations (p. 86). Skepticism about the authenticity of neo-Malthusianism began to grow among researchers and the public during the late 1960s and early 1970s. Birth rates in some developing countries had begun to decline by that time; and the public fear about the possibility of a "population bomb" and massive "famine" steadily diminished. Neo-Malthusian mass organization, such as Zero Population Growth, suffered dramatic reduction in membership as a result.

In discussing the distinct agendas of the second wave feminist movement, Hodgson and Watkins (1997) pointed out the different views among the liberal and radical members with regard to gender equality, population, and women's reproductive health and reproductive rights. For liberal feminists, adequate accessibility to contraception and abortion is essential for women to have control over their family formation, to compete with men in the workplace, to achieve equality in society, and eventually to achieve their reproductive health. Radical feminists, on the other hand, insist that women's reproductive choices should not be sacrificed at the expense of the collective good. Rosalind Petcheky (1990) positioned women's decision to choose within the social context and the sexual power relations between women and men. Petchey (1990) raised the questions: who controls fertility, under what conditions, through what methods, and for what purposes? Petcheky also pointed out that it is the arrangement of the power relations in the division of labor that has a direct influence on women's reproductive freedom and women's reproductive health.

The international women's health movement of the 1970s and the 1980s had its roots in the issue of human rights that emerged in Europe during the 16th century as military interventions sought to punish the states that were found guilty of abusing religious minorities. The effort to abolish the slave trade and to protect the rights of workers throughout the 19th century marked a growing international concern for human rights (Weissbrodt 1988). The ideology of protecting human rights grew significantly in the years following World War I, a war that claimed 20 million lives. The International Committee of the Red Cross was founded in 1869 in Geneva for the purpose of reducing the horror of the war. Human rights concerns after World War I also led to the formation of the League of Nations and the International Labor Organization (ILO) in 1919.

With the horrors of Nazi Germany fresh in mind, the victorious allies came together and created the United Nations in 1945. The Charter of the United

Nations was adopted in the same year. The Preamble of the Charter reaffirmed the "faith in fundamental human rights, in the dignity and worth of the human person, in the equal rights of men and women and of nations large and small," and the determination "to employ international machinery for the promotion of the economic and social advancement of all peoples." (United Nations Office of the High Commissioner for Human Rights – UNHCHR 1945, Charter of the United Nations, Preamble). Three years later in 1948, the United Nations Assembly adopted the Universal Declaration of Human Rights. It is the first international document on human rights. Article One claimed that "All human beings are born free and equal in dignity and rights. They are endowed with reason and conscience and should act toward one another in a spirit of brotherhood." Article Three stated that "Everyone has the right to life, liberty and security of person." Following the adoptions of the United Nations Declaration, a number of human rights instruments were drafted, such as the International Covenant on Economic, Social, and Cultural Rights, the Optional Protocol to the Civil and Political Covenant, the Convention on Political Rights of Women (1952), the Convention on the Nationality of Married Women (1957), and the Convention on the Consent to Marriage, Minimum Age for Marriage and Registration of Marriage (1962). The International Bill of Rights has been accepted by almost all governments in the world as a yardstick by which to measure the degree of respect for and compliance with international human rights standards.[3] A number of other international conventions then followed, including the Convention on the Political Rights of Women (entered into force in 1954), the International Conference on Human Rights (1968 in Teheran), and the International Women's Year World Conference (1975 in Mexico City).

The keystone for the promotion of women's rights, gender equality, and women's reproductive health and well-being in general is the Convention on the Elimination of All Forms of Discrimination against Women (CEDAW 1979).[4] It is known as the international bill of rights for women and considered to be the first comprehensive international legal instrument to address the rights of women, including their right to reproductive choices and reproductive health. The Preamble of the Convention spelled out the responsibilities of "State Parties" to ensure the right to protect the health and safety of women, "including the safeguarding of the function of reproduction" (Article 11.1.f) and the right "to decide freely and

3 The Universal Declaration of Human Rights, the International Covenant on Civil and Political Rights, the International Covenant on Economic, Social, and Cultural Rights, and its two Optional Protocols (Optional Protocol to the International Covenant on Civil and Political Rights, Second Optional Protocol to the International Covenant on Civil and Political Rights) together are called the International Bill of Human Rights. Available at: www.unhchr.ch/html/menu6/2/fs2.htm.

4 In 1966, the United Nations adopted the International Convention on the Elimination of Racial Discrimination. The move to advance women's equality was more prolonged simply because violations of women's rights were not as visible to male authorities as those suffered on racial grounds.

responsibly on the number and spacing of their children and to have access to the information, education and means to enable them to exercise these rights." (Article 16.1.e). It is considered to be the only human rights treaty so far that affirms women's reproductive rights and reproductive health and their equal access to political and public life.[5] In this respect, the Convention on the Elimination of All Forms of Discrimination against Women (CEDAW) has created a legal basis for addressing the issues related to women's rights to reproductive health and health in general.

The international women's health movement during the late 1970s and the1980s has become an increasingly visible player in influencing international population policies. Differing from the notion that individual well-being should be compromised for the sake of the demographic goal of reducing population size especially in developing countries, the international women's health movement claimed that every woman has the right to have control over her body, her sexuality, and her reproductive life. The movement strongly criticized the failure of the government and international organizations to address women's reproductive health and their status in the family and society. It also questioned the rationale that government-sponsored population policies have been used for achieving demographic goals of reducing population size. The movement grew substantially in both numbers and political strength during the last two decades. A central tenet of the movement was that women's reproductive health and their health in general, not the macro-demographic objectives, are of paramount concern (García-Moreno and Claro 1994).

A number of international and regional organizations have been involved in the advocacy and networking effort of the international women's health movement, such as the Convention on the Elimination of All Forms of Discrimination against Women (CEDAW), Development Alternatives with Women for a New Era (DAWN), Women Watch, the United Nations Joint Programme on HIV/AIDS (UNAIDS), and the United Nations Children's Fund (UNICEF). During the late 1980s and the 1990s, the United Nations organized a number of international conferences and conventions and adopted many legal instruments to promote gender equality and to improve women's reproductive health, for instance, the Third World Conference on Women (1985), the World Conference on Human Rights (1993), the 10th International Women and Health Meeting (1995), and the World Summit for Social Development (1995). In 1994, the International Conference on Population and Development (ICPD) was held in Cairo, Egypt and adopted the Programme of Action. The Cairo document reflected two main trends. First, women's reproductive health is important in its own right. Women are not just mothers of their children; they are important and valuable members of the society. Second, women's reproductive health should not be understood as only a biological process. It is, instead, deeply imbedded in the social, economic,

---

5 Countries that have ratified or acceded to the Convention are legally bound to put its provisions into practice. They are also committed to submit national reports, at least every four years, on measures they have taken to comply with their treaty obligations.

and political environment (Pillai and Wang 1999, Sadik 2000, Sen, George, and Östlin 2002). Differing from the conventional demographic perspectives on health, the Programme of Action called for reducing infant, child, and maternal mortality and expanding the access to education, particularly for girls. The Cairo document affirmed that gender equality and the integration of human rights and nondiscrimination laws are the precondition for women to attain reproductive health and that women's reproductive health status is closely related to economic development and the enhancement of women's human rights and gender equality (Klitsch 1999, Chatterjee and Riley 2001, Wang and Pillai 2001). At the Cairo Conference, the Prime Minister of Norway, Gro Harlem Brundtland, openly challenged the moral base of the anti-abortion stance, claiming that "Morality becomes hypocrisy if it means accepting mothers suffering or dying in connection with unwanted pregnancies and illegal abortions and unwanted children living in misery." (quoted from *New York Times*, September 6, 1994: A1, A9).

The United Nations Fourth World Conference on Women (1995) reaffirmed the international commitment to women's reproductive health through the improvement of gender equality and sustainable development. The Conference reiterated women's rights to "the enjoyment of the highest attainable standard of physical and mental health," (Platform for Action, C. 89). It also agreed upon the actions to be taken in its five strategic objectives: (1) Increase women's access through life cycle to appropriate, affordable, and quality health care, information and related services; (2) Strengthen preventive programs that promote women's health; (3) Undertake gender-sensitive initiatives that address sexually transmitted diseases, HIV/AIDS, and sexual and reproductive health issues; (4) Promote research and disseminate information on women's health; and (5) Increase resources and monitor follow-up for women's health. The Millennium Development Goals (MDGs) of the United Nations adopted in 2001 represented a global effort to reduce poverty, infant and maternal mortality, to promote gender equality and education especially for girls, and to combat HIV/AIDS. The Women's Global Network for Reproductive Rights (WGNRR) held its 2005 conference in India. According to WGNRR, women's reproductive rights and reproductive health include good quality comprehensive reproductive health services that meet women's needs; safe and effective contraception and sterilization; safe and legal abortion; safe pregnancy and childbirth; safe and effective treatment for the causes of infertility; and freedom from population policies and social codes that pressure some women to have children and others to not have children. The Convention on the Elimination of All Forms of Discrimination Against Women (CEDAW) together with the Programme of Action of the 1994 International Conference on Population and Development (ICPD), the Platform for Action of the 1995 Beijing Fourth World Conference on Women, and the ten-year review of the Platform for Action in May 2005 have provided the global and fundamental blueprint for improving women's reproductive health through global efforts to combat social injustice and to strengthen gender equality (Birn 1999, Klitsch 1999, Chatterjee and Riley 2001). In addition, the International Women's Health Coalition (IWHC) has helped to revolutionize the way the world views population policies by putting the needs and rights of women first and stressing the centrality of reproductive health services.[6] Sen and Grown (1987) pointed out that international and women's organizations have made substantial influence on the policy processes and played a strategic role in promoting gender equality and advancing women's reproductive health worldwide.

According to Higer (1995), there were basically two strategies within the international women's health movement. The first strategy is considered to be a reformist strategy. This strategy called for a reproductive health approach to family planning and population stabilization. The alternative strategy was of a more radical view. Advocates of the alternative view claimed that current family planning programs tend to be coercive and that women's reproductive health and reproductive rights are important in themselves rather than a means to achieving the demographic goals and objectives.

Influenced by the international women's health movement, Allan Rosenfield and Deborah Maine (1985) began to look at what is called the maternal child field (MCH) and asked the questions: "Where is the M in MCH?" and why so little attention is being given to the health of the mother in maternal and child health programs in developing countries. They called for a major investment in a system of comprehensive maternity care. Dawn (1987) declared that "Control over reproduction is a basic need and a basic right for all women. Linked as it is to women's health and social status, as well as to the powerful social structures of religion, state control and administrative inertia, and private profit, it is from the perspective of poor women that this right can best be understood and affirmed." (quoted from Sen and Grown 1987: 49).

Mann (1997) and Mann Gostin, Gruskin, Brennan, Lazzarini, and Fineberg (1999) proposed three interconnected theoretical principles regarding the gender equality approach to health and reproductive health in particular. The first is based on the observation that violations of gender equality have negative impact on the physical, mental, and social well-being of the population especially on women's reproductive health outcomes. The second principle is based on the proposition that the enhancement of gender equality in society appears to broaden the choices women (and men) have in terms of improving the well-being and health status of the overall population as well as women's reproductive health. The third principle focuses on health policies, programs, and practices. Certain public health policies, such as prioritization of certain health issues and restricted rights to health of a subpopulation may ruin human rights including women's human rights. Mann and the colleagues (2000) pointed out that while these principles are already

6 IWHC was founded in 1984 by Joan Dunlop and Adrienne Germain. By 1994, IWHC had won an unprecedented international consensus at the 1994 International Conference on Population and Development. There, governments agreed that women's reproductive health, their empowerment, and their human rights must be global priorities.

well documented, they require further elaboration and additional analysis and exploration.

The gender equality approach to reproductive health thus implies that women have the right to reproductive self determination and reproductive health care as well as the obligations of the state to provide women with the access to social, economic, and political resources in the community and the society as a whole (Center for Reproductive Rights – CRLP 2000). The right to reproductive self determination includes the right to plan one's own family,[7] the right to freedom from interference in reproductive decision making,[8] and the right to be free from all forms of violence and coercion that affect one's sexual and reproductive life.[9] The right to reproductive health care is rooted in the provisions of international human rights instruments, including the Universal Declaration of Human Rights (United Nations Doc. A/810. 1948) and the International Covenant on Economic, Social, and Cultural Rights (Art. 12, 993 U.N.T.S. 3., 1976). The right to reproductive health is also recognized by the Convention on the Elimination of All forms of Discrimination against Women (CEDAW 1979). The principle of the reproductive rights and the equal rights of women and men is contained in the Charter of the United Nations, the Universal Declaration of Human Rights and all subsequent major international human rights instruments.

Cook (1995) argued that women's reproductive health fits within a social framework of gender equality. Although differences in health care needs between women and men do exist in relation to biological and physiological differences, it does not automatically justify health inequalities in society (Sen, George, and Ostlin 2002). In this sense, the gender equality approach recognizes that women's reproductive health is not merely a medical matter; therefore, it cannot be separated from the gender-based power relations that systematically disadvantage women and girls. Malhotra and Mehra (1999) pointed out that the gender equality approach calls attention to women's access to and their control over economic, social and human resources essential for creating the conditions for women to achieve

7 The Final Act of the International Conference on Human Rights, Teheran, 1968 defined the right to plan one's own family as the rights of the "parents" "to determine freely and responsibly the number and spacing of their children and the right to adequate education and information in this respect." The Report of the United Nations World Population Conference (Bucharest 1974) changed "parents" into "all couples and individuals" who "have the basic human rights to determine freely and responsibly the number and spacing of their children and have the information, education, and means to do so; and the responsibility of couples and individuals in the exercise of this right takes into account the needs of their living and future children, and their responsibilities toward the community."

8 The right to freedom from interference in reproductive decision making is often referred to as the right to bodily autonomy and physical integrity.

9 The right to be free from all forms of violence and coercion is stated in the Report of the International Conference on Population and Development (1994). Reproductive rights "also include the right to make decisions concerning reproduction free of discrimination, coercion and violence, as expressed in human rights documents."

reproductive health goals and improve their reproductive health outcomes. Cook (1995) has reminded us that in many parts of the world, due to legal and customary practices, women still lack access to economic and social resources. Women are still facing systematic and persistent denial of equal opportunities in their families and the community. In many parts of the world today especially in developing countries, the existing hierarchical ordering embedded within the social, economic and political systems still reflects female inferiority and male dominance. Basu (2000) argued that the gender equality approach can provide a new and sensitive way of interpreting demographic processes. Langermann and Niebrugge-Brantley (1992) explicated the gender equality approach in the following way:

> First, its major 'object' for investigation, the starting point of all its investigations, is the situation (or the situations) and experiences of women in society. Second, it treats women as the central 'subjects' in the investigative process; that is, it seeks to see the world from the distinctive vantage point (or vantage points) of women in the social world. Third, feminist theory is critical and activist on behalf of women, seeking to produce a better world for women – and thus, it argues, for humankind. (Langermann and Niebrugg-Brantley 1992: 447)

According to Langermann and Niebrugge-Brantley, the gender equality approach is women centered. Sen (1994) and McDaniel (1996, 2002) claimed that a women-centered gender equality approach is a necessary precondition to the study of demographic and social phenomena and that social scientists can make substantial contributions to this endeavor.

To put women at the center of the analysis, Dunn, Almquist, and Chafetz (1993) suggested adding such variables as (1) which sex gets how much of what socially valued and scarce resources and (2) what features of social structure create this sex-based distribution of resources. Haney (2000), meanwhile, introduced a feminist state perspective that identifies the role of the state patriarchy to shape women's experiences and gender relations through legal codes, penal policies, and welfare provision. This implies that the state has both the legal and the moral responsibility to protect and promote reproductive health and the matters related to social and economic justice for women. The women-centered gender equality approach, therefore, questions the liberal conception of the state as a neutral and benign instrument and the Marxist notion that the state serves only the class interest in capitalistic societies. The gender equality approach, in this regard, offers a direct critique of the structural functionalist perspective that society is composed of interrelated parts that work harmoniously for the maintenance of the whole. Central to this macro-level understanding of gender equality is the notion that social arrangements and constraints reflect the processes of the hierarchal control over women's life experiences, their sexuality, and reproductive health.

For that reason, the most important precondition for women to achieve reproductive health is a socioeconomic and political environment where women are able to acquire their claims to reproductive health and well-being and the control over the circumstances under which they live (Dixon-Mueller 1993, Orloff 1993, Cook 1995, Howard 1995, Sen, George, and Ostlin 2002). Many in the population field have begun to realize that population health related programs and policies that ignore women's concerns and experiences will be ineffective over the long term. Mann (1966, 1997) and Gostin (2000) pointed out that the gender equality approach has provided a useful framework for understanding and analyzing the social structural roots of reproductive health and the obligations of the state government to implement social policies that provide women with equal opportunities for a wide variety of economic, political, and social resources.

Sen, George, and Ostlin (2002), in their book *Engendering International Health*, raised the question: how and to what extent gender equality is important to the consideration of the causes of women's health and their reproductive health in particular. They reminded us that the gender equality analysis of health and women's reproductive health that emerged from its infancy in the late 1990 has yet to mature into a perspective that will eventually influence the mainstream thinking in international health. Lincoln Chen (2002), at the same time, clearly stated that reproductive health disparities, especially with regard to gender, are likely to remain one of the premier health challenges of the 21st century.

Chapter 2
Theoretical Explanations of the Proposed Model

Chapter 2 focuses on the conceptual framework and the theoretical explanations of the proposed model. The proposed model explores the impact of women's rights, gender equality, and maternal and child care on women's reproductive health with economic and political development as the background factors.

There are nine sections in this chapter and each section represents one of causal flows specified in the path diagram of the proposed model. The first section focuses on the conceptual framework of women's rights and perspectives to explain the relationship between women's rights and women's reproductive health. Section two provides discussions on the conceptual framework of gender equality and theoretical explanations of the relationship between gender equality and women's reproductive health. Section three focuses on perspectives to explain the relationship between maternal-child care and women's reproductive health. Section four provides discussions on the relationship between economic development and gender equality. Section five focuses on the relationship between political development and gender equality. Section six provides discussions on perspectives to explain the relationship between economic development and women's rights. Section seven deals with the relationship between political development and women's rights. Section eight focuses on theoretical perspectives to explain the relationship between economic development and maternal-child care; and section nine provides discussions with regard to the relationship between political development and maternal-child care.

2.1 Women's Human Rights and Reproductive Health

I. Conceptualizing Human Rights and Women's Rights

Human Rights as Natural Rights in the Western Tradition and the Women Question The origins of the human rights concept in the Western tradition could be traced back to the political and natural law philosophy of the European Enlightenment and the intellectual heritage of Thomas Hobbes (1588–1679),[1] John

1 Hobbes lived in a time of social and political turmoil in England. The society was divided religiously, economically, and by region. Hobbes saw society as a market place dominated by contractual exchanges. Two points are apparent in his state of nature theory.

Locke (1632–1704),[2] and Jean Rousseau (1712–1778).[3] Central to the natural law philosophy is the belief that man has the capacity to "reason' and is thus entitled to individual liberty and inalienable rights. The modern philosophical justification for individual rights is grounded in the doctrine of liberalism, particularly in the work of Immanuel Kant (1724–1804). Kant (1788) wrote in his *Second Critique* that human beings ought to be treated with respect as an end in itself, not as a means to another person's end. The basis for such respect lies in the fact that human beings have the potential for reason and moral actions. Critics of the natural law philosophy, such as Edmunde Burke (1729–1797), David Hume (1711–1776), and Jeremy Bentham (1748–1832), opposed the abstract premises of natural law and called for secular moral theories and the protection of individual freedoms and entitlements by written laws. For instance, Jeremy Bentham, in his *Introduction to the Principles of Morals and Legislation* (1780) provided an analysis of the distinction between individual hedonic calculation (maximizing individual utility) and social hedonic calculation. He articulated its basic foundations of utilitarianism as:

> Nature has placed mankind under the governance of two sovereign masters, pain and pleasure. It is for them alone to point out what we ought to do as well as to determine what we shall do. On the one hand, the standard of right and wrong, on the other, the chain of causes and effects, are fastened to their throne. (Bentham 1780: 1)

For Bentham, analyses and decisions are judged by their effect on the sum total of people's well-being rather than by individual choices and rights.

First, in the state of nature (state of human beings without civil society), human beings have the right to do whatever they think necessary to ensure their self preservation and to judge what will ensure their self preservation. In the state of nature, Hobbes argued that there is no agreed-upon authority to decide if human beings are right or wrong and that they each have a right to all things, "even to one another's body." (*Leviathan* xiv.4). Hobbes' second argument concerns the danger posed by our differences in judgments of what is right or wrong.

2 One of John Lock's intellectual interest centered on the nature of the self. In his *Two Treatises of Government* (1690), Locke refuted the theory of absolute sovereignty of the Monarch and the doctrine of the divine put forward by Robert Filmer (1680) and argued for the independence of the individual person. He wrote that the state of nature knows no government and that men are born free and equal in rights and are entitled to natural rights including the right to life, liberty, and property.

3 Jean-Jacques Rousseau was one of the most influential thinkers during the Enlightenment. In his second essay *Discourse on the Origin of Inequality among Men*, although not well received by his contemporaries in the academic community, Rousseau saw human beings as free agents. Rousseau (1762) outlined in his book tiled *The Social Contract* how a government can coexist in such a way that it protects the equality and character of its citizens.

The American Declaration of Independence (1776) affirmed the inalienable right to life, liberty, and the pursuit of happiness. Following the French Revolution, the Declaration of the Rights of Man and the Citizen (August 26, 1789) laid out 17 articles in which the will of the King as the source of governing authority was replaced by the protection of natural rights (Appendix B. Declaration of the Rights of Man and the Citizen, 26 August 1789). The Declaration brought together two streams of thought: one springing from the Anglo-American tradition of legal and constitutional guarantees of individual liberties,[4] and the other from the Enlightenment's belief that reason should guide all human affairs.

However, the natural rights in the Declarations do not hold true for women, or religious minorities, or men who did not own property or slaves. Writers, philosophers, and social scientists have long debated about women's rights in society and argued that the natural law philosophy is neglectful of women's rights and their status in society and within the family. Simone de Beauvoir (1949) wrote in *The Second Sex* that "… humanity is male and man defines woman not in herself but as relative to him; she is not regarded as an autonomous being." (p. xviii).

Condorcet (1790) raised the question of women's political rights and argued for complete equality between women and men. Condorcet wrote that "It would be difficult to prove that women are incapable of exercising the right of citizenship. Why should beings exposed to pregnancies and to passing indispositions not be able to exercise rights that no one ever imagined taking away from people who have gout every winter or who easily catch cold?" (p. 120). One year later in 1791, Olympe de Gouges (1748–1793) issued the Declaration of the Rights of Women in which Gouges declared that "Women are born free and remain equal to man in rights. Social distinctions may be based only on common utility." (p. 125).

Human Rights as Social Entitlement The development of socialism in the 19th century expanded the concept of human rights as natural rights to include not only the right to be free from state interventions but also the right to have the state redress economic inequalities (Pillai and Wang 1999). The premise of human rights as a social entitlement implied that the state has the responsibility to guarantee freedom and opportunities for all of its citizens, and more importantly, to assure certain entitlements to all persons (Dixon-Mueller 1993). These entitlements are often called economic and social rights, or welfare rights. These social entitlements include the right to an adequate standard of living, the right to education and work, the right to just and favorable work conditions, and the right to the protection against unemployment without distinction of race, color, sex, language, religion, or national and social origin (United Nations 2002). Note that the philosophical origins of human rights as social entitlement in developing

4 The Anglo-American tradition of legal guarantees of rights dated back to the Magna Carta or "Great Charter" of 1215. In it, King John of England guaranteed certain liberties to the free men of his Kingdom. In 1628, the English Parliament drew up the *Petition of Rights* restating the "rights and liberties of the subjects."

countries differed from those in developed countries, especially during the period of colonization. The current recognition of human rights as social entitlements in developing countries is in part due to their membership in the global entities such as the United Nations.

The ideology of human rights as social entitlement grew significantly in the years following World War II. The Universal Declaration of Human Rights adopted in 1948 was considered to have provided the most comprehensive principles of human rights and non-discrimination. Article 1 declared that "All human beings are born free and equal in dignity and rights." Article 2 affirmed that "Everyone is entitled to all the rights and freedoms set forth in this Declaration, without distinction of any kind, such as race, color, sex, language, religion, political or other opinion, national or social origin, property, birth or other status." Article 3 stated that "Everyone has the right to life, liberty and security of person." Article 25 affirmed that "Everyone has the right to standard of living adequate for the health and well-being of himself and of his family, including food, clothing, housing and medical care, necessary social services, and the right to security in the event of unemployment, sickness, disability, widowhood, old age or other lack of livelihood in circumstances beyond control."

Two multilateral international conferences were later convened to implement the principles of the Declaration; one was on civil and political rights, and the other on social and economic rights. Article 1 of the International Covenant on Civil and Political Rights declared that all persons have the right to choose their political status and to pursue their economic, social, and cultural interest. It further asserted that the state parties have the responsibilities to promote the realization of the right of self determination of all persons. The International Covenant on Economic, Social, and Cultural Rights required that ratifying nations should guarantee fair wages and equal remuneration for equal work, equal promotion opportunities, safe and healthful working conditions, and reasonable limitations of working hours. It also called on ratifying nations to assure the availability of medical care to all, to make primary education compulsory and secondary and higher education generally available and equally accessible to all.

Beginning in the late 19th century, liberal reformers and feminists proposed that human rights be extended to women. The Commission on the Status of Women (CSW) was established in 1946 as a functional body of the United Nations Economic and Social Council (ECOSOC) for the advancement of women's rights in political, economic, civil, social, and educational fields. It was not until the 1950s that the international community and the United Nations began to address the issues concerning women's human rights and social entitlements. The International Labor Organization (ILO) held a number of conventions that focused on the rights of women (Defeis 1991). The ILO's Convention Concerning Equal Remuneration for Men and Women Workers for Work of Equal Value was held in 1951 and identified equal remuneration as the "rates of remuneration established without discrimination based on sex." (Article 1). Article 2 of ILO's Convention specified that "each member shall, by means appropriate to the methods in operation for determining rates of remuneration, promote and, in so far as in consistent with such methods, ensure the application to all workers of the principle of equal remuneration for men and women for work of equal value." The 1958 Convention Concerning Discrimination further identified discrimination in employment and occupation as "(1) any distinction, exclusion or preference made on the basis of race, color, sex, religion, political opinion, social or national origin, which has the effect of nullifying or impairing equality of opportunity or treatment in employment or occupation and (2) such other distinction, exclusion or preference which has the effect of nullifying or impairing equality of opportunity or treatment in employment or occupation as may be determined by the Member concerned after consultation with representative employers' and workers' organizations, where such exist, and with other appropriate bodies." (Article 1).

Around the same time, the United Nations held four conventions that primarily focused on issues of women's rights. The Convention on the Political Rights of Women (adopted in 1952) identified that women are entitled to vote in all elections on equal terms with men and that women are eligible to serve in all publicly elected bodies without any discrimination. It was the first international law instrument to recognize and protect the political rights of women. The other three conventions represented the first international agreements on women's rights in relation to marriage. The Convention on Nationality of Married Women was adopted in 1957 and stipulated that the separation or dissolution of marriage does not affect the nationality of the wife. The Convention on the Consent to Marriage, Minimum Age for Marriage and Registration of Marriage (adopted in 1962) and the Recommendation on Consent to Marriage, Minimum Age for Marriage and Registration on Marriage (adopted in 1965) reaffirmed that all marriages must be based on free consent of both parties and that no marriage can be entered into by any person under the legally specified age.

The 1960s and 1970s saw the emergence of greater awareness of discrimination against women in many parts of the world and the rise of international women's movements committed to combating it. In the wake of Boserup's (1970) influential study on women's role in economic development, the Convention for the Elimination of All Forms of Discrimination against Women (CEDAW) was adopted in 1979 by a vote of 130 member states with 10 absents. As often referred to as the international women's bill of rights, it is the most comprehensive international legal instrument to date in defining internationally accepted principles on the human rights of women and on the responsibilities of the government "to ensure the full development and advancement of women for the purpose of guaranteeing them the exercise and enjoyment of human rights and fundamental freedoms on the basis of equality with men." (Article 3). Article 12 insisted that state parties take appropriate measures to eliminate discrimination against women in the fields of health care in order to ensure, on the basis of equality of men and women, their access to health care services, including those related to family planning, pregnancy and the postnatal care, and adequate nutrition during pregnancy and lactation. Currently, 185 countries, over 90 percent of the members of the United Nations, have ratified the treaty.

Six years after the adoption of the Convention for the Elimination of All Forms of Discrimination against Women (CEDAW), the Third World Conference on Women held in Nairobi adopted the Nairobi Forward Looking Strategies for the Advancement of Women. In 1995, the Fourth World Conference on Women held in Beijing, China reaffirmed, in its Platform for Action, that women's human rights are part of the universal human rights and social justice and called for (1) access of women to political structures at all levels and equal political empowerment at all decision-making levels, (2) recognition, protection, compensation, financial and other assistance and full legal status for millions of women and children and the victims of nuclear and other environmental catastrophes, (3) universally accessible, high quality, non-discriminatory health care to sponsor and support women-controlled research for the prevention and cure of HIV/AIDS, to prohibit any forms of discrimination of women with HIV/AIDS, and to ensure women's access to information, care, support, and treatment of HIV/AIDS, (4) the development and sustained use of affirmative action by both the private and public sectors of society to ensure the equality of women, (5) all the media to change the present negative, exploitive, and sexualized images of women and children to positive ones, (6) a reshaping of education for all children, beginning at the primary levels, to sensitize them about human rights, gender issues, and non-violent conflict resolution, stressing the need for world peace, (7) full implementation of the UN Decade for Human Rights Education and the prevention of human rights violations against women, and (8) new and additional financial, technical, and other resources to successfully implement the plans and commitments from the Nairobi, Rio de Janeiro, Vienna, Cairo, Copenhagen, and Beijing conferences and member states to fulfill their obligations under the Convention on the Elimination of All Forms of Discrimination against Women. Since the passage of the Platform for Action, follow-up reviews and a number of other international efforts have further contributed toward identifying issues of women's human rights as social entitlement, including women's economic, social, and political rights.

Human Rights in Sociological Theories The synthetic philosophy of Herbert Spencer (1820–1903) on anti-government individualism takes moral rights seriously. Spencer (1884) claimed in his book *The Man Versus the State* that basic moral rights are natural rights and that the social whole exists only to facilitate the welfare of its members. For Spencer, the corporate life of the society must be subservient to the lives of its members, and not vice versa. Therefore, an important function of the government is to protect the unmolested pursuit of happiness of its members. Spencer saw society as a super organic substance organized as a social entity in the same way that a living organism is organized as a biological entity. Individuals in society, while competing for space, food, and shelter, move either toward decay or higher states of perfection.

Emile Durkheim (1858–1917) turned Spencer's anti-government individualism around, arguing that society cannot be derived from the propensity of individuals to trade and barter in order to maximize their own happiness and that people do not trade and barter at random, but that they tend to follow a framework of normative controls and social regulations. Durkheim (1893, 1897) saw men as creatures whose desires are unlimited and argued that the preservation of norms is essential for achieving solidarity and integration in society. Durkheim's legal theory focused on law as a social control factor and as an "external" index in the complex moral fabrics of social life to help maintain collective morality. Law, according to Durkheim, is the organization of social life in its most stable and precise form. In well regulated societies, laws as a form of social control set limits on individual propensities so that "each in his sphere vaguely realizes the extreme limits on individual propensities" and "each in his sphere vaguely realizes the extreme limits set to his ambitions and aspires to nothing beyond." (Durkheim 1897: 255). When social regulations break down, Durkheim stated, the controlling influence of society on individual propensities is no longer effective and individuals are left to their own devices. Durkheim called such a state of affairs an "anomie," a property of the social structure that is characterized by greater or lesser normative regulations.

Durkheim reacted against the atomistic drift of most Enlightenment philosophy and grounded his sociological thought on a concern for the maintenance of social order. In *The Division of Labor in Society* (1893), Durkheim described the rights of individuals in terms of morality, obligations, and sanctions. He distinguished between two types of societies, mechanical and organic. Mechanical solidarity is characterized by a relatively undifferentiated social structure in which there is little or no division of labor. Due to the increase in spatial concentration of people and the number and efficacy of the means of communications among people, society becomes more sophisticated and complex in terms of the division of labor. Durkheim called the more advanced and complex society "organic solidarity." In organic societies, morality and collective conscious are rooted in the interdependence and formal relations among the members of the society. In organic societies, members are less alike compared with those in mechanic societies. For Durkheim, modern societies contain the potentialities for individualism within social regulations.

Karl Marx (1818–1883) and Frederick Engels (1820–1895), unlike Durkheim and Spencer, were highly critical of the principles of rights that emerged from the French Revolution (Sjoberg and Vaughan 1993). Marx (1848) rejected natural rights and saw those rights as a bourgeois invention. In his economic analysis of capitalism, Marx associated the rights of the individuals to their social class status and the ownership of the means of production. Under the capitalistic system, the proletariat is exposed to all forms of economic exploitation and they are the prey of the bourgeois conspiracy. Marx used the term "alienation" to refer to the inconsistency in the lives of the working-class people in terms of their human nature and the labor they are doing as a result of the antagonistic relationship between the bourgeoisie and the proletariat. The proletariat has no country. In their lives, laws, religion, and morality symbolize nothing but bourgeois prejudice. Women of the working class reproduce to supply the capitalists with a cheap labor force. According to Marx, communism provides every member of the society with equal rights and freedom. Under a communist society, each contributes according to their ability and receives according to their needs.

Max Weber (1864–1920), however, believed that individuals in modern societies are incapable of resisting the iron cage of bureaucratic life. The "steel-hard cage" of the modern and bureaucratic instrumentalism is, in large part, escape proof and nobody can evade the possibility of being a cog in a bureaucratic machine and a cheerful robot (Mills 1961). Weber (1921) wrote that rational calculation "reduces every worker to a cog in this bureaucratic machine and sending himself in this light, he will merely ask how to transform himself into somewhat a bigger cog." (p. iii). According to Weber, bureaucracy in modern societies is characterized by a complex division of labor, a conception of rationality, and a hierarchy of authority and power. A very important sociological question Weber asked was that of the role of power and authority in confining the individual person's freedom of choice.[5] Weber maintained that in modern societies, the state establishes "a monopoly of the legitimate use of physical force in the enforcement of its order" to secure its privileged positions (p. 154). Freedom of choice and individual rights are only between bureaucracy and dilettantism in the field of administration.

According to Weber (1904–05), modern societies provide individuals with more leisure time and material comfort as a result of scientific and technological advancement. Freedom of choice is a result of activities and decisions arising from informed choices. Large-scale organizations in modern societies function to undermine human rights. Human values and freedoms serve as the means to achieve efficiency, calculability, and predictability of the organizations. Mean-end rationality and value rationality are mechanisms for individuals to achieve personal goals. Weber described individual rights under a capitalistic system as "an immense cosmos into which the individual is born, and which presents itself to him, at least as an individual, insofar as he is involved in the system of market relationships, to conform to capitalist rules of action." (p. 54).

According to Talcott Parsons (1902–1979), the basic unit of the social system is the "status-role." Parsons (1951) defined the social system in terms of its normative structure and he believed that human action can adapt to the needs of the society through four functional imperatives: adaptation (A), goal attainment

5 Weber in his book *Economy and Society* (1921) presented three types of authority, traditional, charismatic, and rational-legal. Traditional authority that predominates in pre-modern societies is based on the belief in the sanctity of tradition and in particular persons who may either inherit it or be invested with it by a higher authority. Charismatic authority rests on the appeal of leaders who claim allegiance because of their extraordinary virtuosity, whether ethical, heroic, or religious. Rational-legal authority is characterized by the hierarchical relations in modern societies and it is anchored in impersonal rules that have been legally enacted or contractually established.

(G), integration (I), and latency (pattern maintenance) (L). The AGIL action scheme functions at all levels of the social, cultural, and personality systems and behavioral organisms. Individuals perform their AGIL action by means of their adaptation to the subsystems of economy, polity, the fiduciary system, and the societal community. Their need-dispositions can be satisfied under the constraints of social control and individual conformity.[6] Parsons identified three types of need-dispositions. The first type impels actors to seek love and approval from social relationships. The second type includes internalized values and norms that lead actors to conform to cultural and social expectations. The third type is role expectations that lead actors to give and receive appropriate responses. Parsons' structural functionalism that is based on the AGIL scheme characterizes the "freedom of human action" as being circumscribed by the social structure and internalized by human adaptive skills.

Based on Weber's bureaucratic structure theory and Parsons' AGIL action scheme, Sjoberg and Vaughan (1993) recognized four systems of bureaucratic structure within the global context that affect the freedom of choice of individuals. The first system consists of organizations with finance capital that can shape the economic, political, and cultural orientations of the nation-states. The second system involves large-scale bureaucratic structures that have emerged in the form of technological, scientific, and educational complex. The importance of these organizations signifies the fact that the modern economic system depends on scientific innovations. The third type of the system refers to the mass media that serve to shape the nature of public opinions. The fourth system is related to the production of goods. Sjoberg and Vaughan considered the rights of the individual to be influenced by these four systems of bureaucratic organizations.

Classical and contemporary sociological theories have broadly touched on the issue of human rights. Sociology, unlike history and anthropology, has not undergone a conceptual transformation in understanding human rights, especially the rights of women (Kandal 1988, Collins and Makowsky 1993). Economically centered models and social class still occupy a central position in the mainstream sociological theories of stratification and human rights (Stacey and Thorne 1985, Ferree and Hall 1996, Chafetz 1997). In Kandal's (1988) words, sociology is faulted for its exclusion of women in most of its subject matters and methodological inquiries. Recently, as Pearce (2001) pointed out, sociology as an academic discipline lags behind other disciplines in applying itself to the human rights debates.

---

6 Parsons (1951) differentiated need-dispositions from drives. The former is the most significant units of motivation of action. The latter is the physiological energy that makes the action possible. That is, need-dispositions are drives that are shaped by the social setting and acquired through the process of action itself, while the drive is part of the biological organism.

II. Perspectives to Explain the Relationship between Women's Human Rights and Reproductive Health

According to Correa and Petchesky (1994), women's human rights have generally been neglected and the Bill of Rights has faulted for its lack of gender sensitivity and its failure to address the relationship between women's reproductive health and women's human rights. Between the late 1960s and early 1980s, concerns over the adverse effects of rapid population growth on economic development and environmental degradation, especially in developing countries became one of the hot topics in academic research and within the international community. Two influential publications both in 1968 delivered a frightening and disastrous picture as a result of rapid population growth. Paul R. Ehrlich wrote in his book titled *The Population Bomb* that:

> The battle to feed all of the humanity is over. In the 1970s and 1980s hundreds of millions of people will starve to death in spite of any crash programs embarked upon now. At this late date, nothing can prevent a substantial increase in the world death rate, although many lives could be saved through dramatic programs to 'stretch' the carrying capacity of the earth by increasing food production. But these programs will only provide a stay of execution unless they are accompanied by determined and successful efforts at population control." Ehrlich predicted that "We are today involved in the events leading to famine; tomorrow we may be destroyed by its consequences. (Prologue)

Echoing Ehrlich, Garrett Hardin (1968) published an article in the journal *Science*, in which Hardin warned of the dilemma of the commons when individuals who act to maximize their own self interest can ultimately destroy a shared and limited resources. Their theory imposed enormous influence on population policies during that time and has prevailed for decades afterwards.

Beginning in the late 1980s, thanks to the women's health movement and international legislations, feminist scholars and social scientists began to question the validity of the neo-Malthusian argument. Among the prominent scholars were Betsy Hartmann (1987), Rebecca Cook (1993, 1995), Susan McDaniel (1996), and Ruth Dixon-Mueller (1998). Their scholarly work has contributed to the current growing visibility of women's reproductive health and human rights. According to Hartmann, Cook, McDaniel, and Dixon-Mueller, population control policies should protect personal integrity, women's reproductive health and their health in general. They further pointed out that the primary obstacles to improving women's reproductive health are rooted in the socioeconomic, legal, and cultural factors of social justice and women's human rights. The World Health Organization (WHO) and the International Women's Health Coalition (IWHC) (1991) made it clear that improvements in women's reproductive health inevitably involve women's rights to have control over their sexuality and reproductive decision making. Correa and Petckesky (1994), Hellsten (2000), and Wickrama and Lorenz (2002) argued for the universal protection of women's human rights as the very basis for the improvement of women's reproductive health around the world. Merali (2000), at the same time, affirmed that reproductive health cannot be promoted without legally binding human rights instruments, such as international and regional human rights treaties and national constitutions. In this study, women's human rights are hypothesized to positively affect women's reproductive health.

2.2 Gender Equality and Women's Reproductive Health

I. Conceptualizing Gender Equality

The issue of gender equality is getting increasing attention in social and political studies (Bradley and Ramirez 1996, Ramirez, Soysal, and Shanahan 1997, Forsythe, Korzeniewicz, and Durrant 2000), and it is becoming an important subject in medical sociology, epidemiology, and interdisciplinary studies of health and illnesses. Gender equality is a particularly sensitive issue, especially in the international and cross-cultural discussions on the status of women relative to that of men.[7] Philosophers have long debated certain moral aspects of women's status in the family and society at large.

The concept of gender emerged during the 1980s as feminist scholars began to question the mainstream sex role theory and recognize the structural basis of gender inequalities. The term gender equality has been widely used among social scientists and policy makers in the international community. For example, the Programme of Action adopted at the 1994 United Nations International Conference on Population and Development (ICDP) devoted a full chapter (Chapter IV) to gender equality and empowerment of women. According to the Programme of Action (1994), gender equality includes providing women with access to employment, income, skill and education information, and elimination of gendered violence in order to achieve reproductive rights and improve reproductive health conditions. The Conference recommended that governments should make changes in the social, cultural, and economic spheres. In its 1999 review of the ICPD implementation, the United Nations General Assembly called for redoubled action to redress gender equality and to eliminate harmful practices, attitudes, and discrimination against women and girls, including zero tolerance among the public for son preference, unequal care for or valuing of girl children, and all forms of violence directed against women, such as female genital mutilation (FGM), rape, incest,

7 Note that the term "gender equity" has been used by some researchers and policy makers. For example, Sen Gita, Asha George, and Prioska Ostlin (2002), in their edited book *Engendering International Health: The Challenge of Equity* used the term gender equity to explain health disparities between women and men. In this book, I prefer to use the term gender equality (or inequality) to imply parity (or disparity) in social, economic, and political outcomes between women and men.

sexual violence, and trafficking. At the Millennium Summit in September 2000, world leaders adopted the UN Millennium Development Goals (MDGs), three of the eight goals aim at promoting gender equality, reducing child mortality, and reducing maternal mortality. Although the ICPD Programme of Action (1994, 2004), the Beijing Platform of Action (1995), and the UN Millennium Declaration (2000a, b) have all reiterated the international obligations to the advancement of women's reproductive health through gender equality, the conceptual framework has remained largely a goal in theory and has not been fully conceptualized nor has it been adequately operationalized (Malhotra and Hehra 1999, Wang 2004, 2007).

Given the obscurity, generally speaking, there are three broad types of mechanisms to explain gender equality (or gender inequality): biological determinism, socialization theory, and the social structural perspective. Biological explanations attribute gender differences to different biological functions. Studies on the hormone-brain-behavior system, for example, emphasize the differences between females and males in the levels of hormone, brain sizes, and the asymmetry and functionality of the two halves of the brain (Hutt 1976, Lynn 1994, Ankney 1995, Monroe 1996, Yoder 1999). In explaining male aggressiveness, Weitz (1977) argued that sex hormones may have a direct effect on the aggressiveness in males and passivity in females and that human socialization practices simply follow the lines of natural hormones. Research findings, however, have been inconsistent. For instance, the left hemisphere of the brain was originally thought to be the locus of reason and intellect and the right hemisphere, the passion and instinct. So males were said to be more left-brained. By the 1970s, brain researchers had found something different, that is, the right brain is the repository of talent, creativity, and genius. So suddenly, males became right brained. Studies on the way females and males use their brains have discovered more within-group variations than between-group variations. That is, there is a much greater difference among females and among males than there is between females and males (Hyde, Fennema, and Laman 1990). Based on the research on primates, Udry (1995) argued that the differences in behavior between the male and the female result from hormonal processes and that the same hormonal processes also cause within-sex differences. More assertive and aggressive females may have a higher testosterone level than less aggressive females; and the same is true for males.

The socialization theory sees gender differences as a product of socialization processes. George Herbert Mead (1934), and Charles Horton Cooley (1902, 1909) viewed social reality as socially and culturally constructed. Socialization theories, such as social learning theory, cognitive development theory, and identification theory explain how individuals develop appropriate behavior through social interactions and become engendered in ways that are defined as socially normative. The socialization theory was called into question recently by feminist scholars, who claimed that if we think of gender differences only in terms of a learned choice, we then overlook the patterns of institutionalized practices that shape our access to economic, social, and political resources and further generate gender inequality.

Following this line of reasoning, socialization serves only as a means to transmit culture and social expectations and affects how women and men choose among options, but it misses the institutional basis of gender inequality that determines which options women and men can choose among.

The third explanation sees gender as a major organizing principle in all of the social systems, including politics, economy, work, education, law, and families. The social structural theories emphasize societal forces that shape gender relations (Blumberg 1984, 1989, Chafetz 1990, 1997, Collins, Chafetz, Blumberg, Coltrane, and Turner 1993, Ebaugh and Chafetz 1999, Cotter, Hermsen, and Vanneman 2001). As Ferree (1990) pointed out, the social construction of maleness and femaleness highlights the unequal social values of women and men in society. That is to say, women and men wield unequal power and opportunities in both relationships and the social organizations of society; and they benefit unequally from the results of social development. As a result, membership in different sex categories may affect the conditions for realizing their full potential to contribute to social, political, and economic development. Karl Marx, Max Weber, C. Wright Mills, Ralf Dahrendorf, and Immanuel Wallerstein are among the mainstream theorists who have made significant contributions in the field.

The social-structural perspectives look at how the control over means of coercion by one sex generates a system of unequal gender relations and gender inequality in society. Gender inequality, according to Chafetz (1990), refers to a gender-based division of labor and power disparity between women and men. Young, Fort, and Danner (1994) considered gender inequality as the departure from parity in the representation of women and men in the key dimensions of the social structure. Rae Lesser Blumberg (1984, 1989) proposed a more Marxian oriented theory that women's control over economic resources relative to men's is a critical variable in explaining gender equality (or inequality) and women's status in the household and the society.

Gender equality (or inequality) is sometimes referred to as women's status, women's empowerment,[8] and female autonomy[9] as it has been suggested by a

8 The word empowerment has also been used in international discussions on issues related to development and women's reproductive health. Yet, it is one of the least understood in terms of how it is to be measured or observed (Medel-Anonuevo 1995).

9 The word autonomy has been used interchangeably with empowerment. Basu and Koolwal (2004) wrote on the conceptual differences between autonomy and empowerment. Autonomy refers to the freedom and liberty to do certain things while empowerment can be defined as the ability to resist control over one's life or to resist the denial of one's rights. Autonomy implies a person's freedom to pursue one's rights and sovereignty. The concept of the freedom to exercise one's rights as authority derived from Rousseau's social contract tradition and Kant's moral philosophy. Dyson and Moore (1983) introduced the concept of female autonomy in an influential paper to explain regional differences in fertility in Northern and Southern India. Their paper and the ones followed soon afterwards have spawned many attempts to define autonomy and to empirically measure the concept. One such scholastic endeavor to define autonomy as liberty, freedom and choice is reflected in

number of social science scholars (German, Nowrojee, and Hnin 1994, Kishor 2000, McDaniel 2002, Smith, Ramakrishnan, Ndiaye, Haddad, and Martorell 2003). Mason (1986) pointed out that in social demography literature, all of these terms, to a large extent, refer to gender equality (or inequality). Gender equality is sometimes interpreted in absolute terms and sometimes relative to men. There is no consensus on a single definition and explanation of the widely employed term, gender equality, although the term has been frequently used by social scientists and policy makers. Recently, feminist scholars and social scientists recognized that the term gender equality is "no unitary," "multidimensional," and "multilevel," rendering it unfeasible to develop a consensus on its definition (Mason 1986, 1993, Sen and Batliwala 2000, Smith, Ramakrishnan, Ndiaye, Haddad, and Martorell 2003).

II. Perspectives to Explain the Relationship between Gender Equality and Women's Reproductive Health

John Stuart Mill (1869) and Charlotte Perkins Gilman (1898) were among the first who wrote on gender equality, women's economic status, and their impact on health. John Stuart Mill noted in *The Subjection of Women* that the subordination of one sex to the other is wrong in itself and that the global oppression of women is the chief hindrances to human improvement and women's health outcomes. Mill argued that the existing social relations between the two sexes ought to be replaced by a principle of perfect equality, admitting no power or privilege on the one side, or disability on the other. Gilman referred to women's subordination and domestic responsibilities, including bearing children, as the "domestic industry of women" (p.14). In this sense, the perception that promoting gender equality is essential for people's health and well-being is not new (Stuart 2000).

In terms of gender equality and its effect on women's reproductive health, early masters of sociological theories were conspicuously quiet (Turner 1998). Human reproduction was considered to be part of the household production. Recent international recognitions of the linkage between health and gender relations began in the United Nations' charters and took form in the Preamble to the 1946 Constitution of the World Health Organization (Easley, Marks, and Morgan 2001, Marks 2001a, b) and a number of international conferences and conventions afterwards (Appendix C. Chronology of International Conferences on Gender Equality, Women's Rights, and Women's Reproductive Health). Mann (1997) proposed two theoretical bases regarding the relationship

---

the work of a number of researchers (e.g., Dixon-Mueller 1998, Jejeenhoy 2000, Malhorra, Schuler, and Boernder 2002, Basu and Koolwal 2004). Autonomy implies that individuals have the capacity to determine events in their own lives through control over resources and information (Bloom, Wypij, and Gupta 2001). Demographic literature on female autonomy for developing countries tends to focus on its instrumental strengths and properties, while literature from developed countries tends to emphasize the value of autonomy as a means of serving women's self interest (England 2000).

between health and gender equality. The first is based on the observation that violations of gender equality have health consequences. The impact of these violations on the physical, mental, and social well-being of women has been adequately documented. The second is that a gender equality approach to public health appears to broaden the choices clients have in terms of improving their health status in general.

Malhotra and Mehra (1999) pointed out that it is women's access to and control over economic, social and human resources that will create the conditions for women to achieve reproductive goals and preferences. Examples of economic resources are income and financial assets. Examples of human resources are education, skills, and knowledge. Social and political resources include membership in social and political groups that directly or indirectly affect decision making in reproductive rights and reproductive health. According to Blumberg (1989), "the greater a woman's relative economic power, the greater the likelihood that fertility pattern will reflect her own perceived utilities and preferences," and "the greater her relative economic power, the greater her control over a variety of other life options, including marriage, divorce, sexuality, …" (p.101). Chafetz (1984, 1988), one of the prominent feminist theorists, argued that the extent to which members in the society have unequal access to the scarce values of their society on the basis of their membership in the sex category[10] and the gender division of labor, by which women are more responsible than men are for the care of infants and young children and for other domestic tasks may perpetuate systems of female disadvantage in achieving reproductive health. In societies where women have little control over social and household resources, they tend to face difficulties in pursuing the need for their own health and much less garnering the self-assurance to act on that need (England 2000, Rosenfield and Schwartz 2005). Growing evidence has shown that the most important precondition for women to achieve reproductive health is a social, economic, and political environment where women are able to acquire their claims to reproductive health and the control over the circumstances under which they live (Hartmann 1987, Dixon-Mueller 1993, Orloff 1993, Howard 1995). A recent study (2008) on the relationship between social and economic status and health outcomes in a national sample of non-institutionalized people aged 52 or over in England suggested that wealth, education, and occupation are related positively to almost all health outcome indicators and it is particularly evident in women.

Sen (1994) argued that the existing social, economic, and political system undermines women's ability to gain social resources and tends to benefit men in two ways. First, structural obstacles restrain women from obtaining social resources. The employment structure, for example, tends to increase women's

10 Scarce values of society include such things as power, material goods, the services of others, prestige-conferring roles, discretionary time, food and medical care, personal autonomy, educational and training opportunities, and safety from physical coercion and assault (Chafetz 1988: 111).

economic dependence on men. Second, gender relations in the family can be affected by women's political and economic status in society. Women's economic dependence on men may prevent them from abandoning oppressive relationships and having better control over their reproductive choices (Bowman 2000).

Gender equality, therefore, may directly affect women's reproductive health independent of fertility decline (Fathalla 1992, Cook 1993, 1995, Dixon-Mueller 1993, Correa and Petchesky 1994, Garcia-Moreno and Claro 1994, Germain, Nowrojee, and Pyne 1994, McDaniel 1996, Yamin 1996, Orubuloye, Oguntimehin, and Sadique 1997, Wagner 1998, Wang and Pillai 2001, Wickrama and Lorenz 2002, Wang 2004).[11] McDaniel (1996, 2002) called for greater attention to women as agents in power relationships in explaining their health status. In this study, gender quality is hypothesized to positively affect women's reproductive health outcomes.

2.3 Maternal-Child Health Care and Women's Reproductive Health

At the 2008 G8 summit meeting, the issue of maternal and child health care was on the agenda and the Partnership for Maternal, Newborn, and Child Health asked the world leaders to increase their spending on maternal and child care and family planning by US$10.2 billion a year. We all know that the earliest days of life are the most vulnerable for a child. Almost 40 percent of under-five mortality takes place during the neonatal period, the first 28 days. The presence of skilled birth attendants at delivery is critical for averting maternal and neonatal mortality (Carlough and McCall 2005). Maternal care is critical for the health of both the mother and her child.

Maternal health care encompasses preconception, prenatal care, and postnatal care, such as contraceptive availability, family planning, and health care during pregnancy and childbirth. In many developing countries, complications of pregnancy and childbirth are the leading causes of deaths among women of reproductive age, causing almost 20 percent of the total burden of disease for women (World Health Organization 2009). A woman in sub-Saharan Africa has a 1 in 16 chance of dying of pregnancy- and childbirth-related causes, compared to 1 in 4,000 women in a developed country (World Health Organization 2006). About 50 percent of the births in developing countries take place without a skilled attendant (United Nations Children's Fund 2004). A large number of studies have indicated that the majority of maternal and infant deaths are associated with the structure and performance of health care services and could be avoided by improving the accessibility and the quality of the reproductive health services

11 A number of studies have found that in societies where women and men enjoy more egalitarian relationships, women appear to enjoy better health outcomes. Note that this notion can not hold true when the overall well-being of the community is jeopardized by events beyond control, such as war or natural disasters.

offered to women (Rosenfield and Maine 1985, Bennett 1997, Castle, Traore, and Cisse 2002, Gottlieb and Lindmark 2002). Substantive evidence especially in clinical studies has shown the importance of maternal-child care in reducing maternal and infant mortality. In this study, a positive relationship between maternal-child care and women's reproductive health is hypothesized.

2.4 Economic Development and Gender Equality

The concept of economic development as a key theme in sociology has its roots in the thought of Comte (1851) and Spencer (1850), and Durkheim's (1893) account of mechanical and organic solidarities. Boserup (1970) defined economic development as a process that accompanies technologically induced economic growth. Economic development goes hand in hand with the reduction in the proportion of the population engaged in agriculture and the increase in the proportion of the population engaged in industry and the service sector. Economic development can be understood as both a process of social differentiation (Durkheim 1893) and ideological diffusion (Castells 1996, Ramirez, Soysal, and Shanahan 1997), and as the transformation in technological and structural conditions (Weber 1947, Mommsen 1974, Luke 1990, Bell 2001). Economic development can be understood as the process of economic advancement as well as social changes as a result of the development of an industrial mode of production. Economic development affects virtually every aspect of society, including physical, social, and the infrastructures involved in production, distribution, and the consumption of services.

The relationship between economic development and gender equality has been the focus of intensive research and theorizing for decades. The economic development approach to gender equality identifies three closely interrelated dimensions, namely economic, e.g, expansion of markets; institutional, e.g., changes in the social structure; and ideological, e.g., changes in the values about gender roles. The relationship between economic development and gender equality has been a much debated issue among social scientists and policy makers (Pedersen 1987, Togunde 1999, Forsythe, Korzeniewicz, and Durrant 2000). The classical economic development theory received criticism in recent years from anthropologists and political scientists for its neglect of the multifarious forms of power relations that exist within and among states (Peterson 2003) and of the cultural factors in the analysis (Castro and Alarcon 2002). The role of cultural convergence and changes in ideological values as a result of economic growth is identified as being more critical than mere economical factors in transforming women's social and economical status (Ramirez, Soysal, and Shanahan 1997, Berkovitch 1999). Castro and Alarcon (2002), however, cautioned the distinction between a causal relationship and a buffer effect of the cultural variables. They found an intervening effect of the cultural variables on the dependent variable.

Despite decades of critique, the theory of economic development still remains dominant in explaining the trajectories of societal development and gender relations (Kahn, Johann, Arnason, Elsenstadt, and Englund 2001). There are mainly four theoretical explanations in the cross-national and development literature. Neoclassical economic theory holds that economic development tends to increase gender equality by providing women with more opportunities for education and paid employment. A number of studies have suggested that gender inequality results primarily from the differences in human capital, such as education, skills, and expected length of labor-force participation (Becker 1985, Clark, Ramsbey, and Adler 1991, Schultz 1997, Bell 2001). To explain the variability in gender equality, neoclassical economic theory suggests more or less linear improvements in women's social and economic status, as either economic growth or the diffusion of ideological egalitarianism promotes gradual enhancement in women's human capital attainment (Weiss, Ramirez, and Tracy 1976, Becker 1985, Norris 1987, Clark 1991, Clark, Ramsbey, and Adler 1991, Clarles 1992, Adler, Boyce, Chesney, Cohen, Folkman, Kahn, and Syme 1994, Castells 1996).[12] These human capital and educational enhancements are in turn expected to contribute to more employment opportunities for women (Bell 2001), and further ideological shifts (Ramirez, Soysal, and Shanahan 1997, Boon 2002). Economic development is likely to disrupt traditional gender role expectations and reengineer cultural values and this shift in attitude is a precursor to gender equality (Inglehart and Norris 2003). Economic development is likely to facilitate certain investment in women by freeing up social resources and opening up opportunities for women in the area of education and labor force participation, which will eventually lead to upward mobility for women and further parity (Pedersen 1987, Thomas 1990, Togunde 1999, Inglehart and Norris 2003). Using the United Nations' measure of gender development index (GDI), a recent cross-national longitudinal study by Forsythe, Korseniewwicz, and Durrant (2000) found a positive and linear relationship between levels of economic development and gender equality.

A second explanation emphasizes the negative impact of the separation of household and economy on gender equality as a result of economic growth (Chatterjee and Riley 2001). The third explanation holds that the relationship between economic development and gender equality is curvilinear (Boserup 1970, Kabeer 1994, Entwisle, Gail, Henderson, Short, and Zhai 1995, Rudd 2000). The fourth explanation focuses on the impact of globalization on gender relations. Much of this research examines the links between the life experiences of women especially those living in developing countries and international rules and financial policies as a result of globalization and international trade. For example, in a research on the effect of globalization on gender relations, Kerr and Sweetman (2003) found that women in developing countries may be

12 Castells (1996) recognized that in the course of globalization and international integration, economic development is more capitalistic in nature and associated with institutional and ideological changes that are part of the free-market capitalism.

pressured by the government to produce cash crops for exports, which may lead to a reduction in women's control over the fruits of their labor. The escalation of trafficking in women is another example that pushes women into forms of precarious transnational employment.

In this study, a linear and positive relationship between economic development and gender equality is hypothesized.

2.5 Political Development and Gender Equality

Concerns over the relationship between political development and gender relations became increasingly prominent in the 1990s (Seidman 1999). Theories on political development mostly focus on the connection between the process of political development and explanatory variables, such as economic development (Lipset 1959, 1960, 1983, Lerner 1968, Sartori 1987, Diamond, Linz, and Lipset 1990, Diamond and Marks 1992), democratic culture and leadership (O'Donnell and Schmitter 1986, Diamond, Linz, and Lipset 1988–9, Fossedal 1989, Sorensen 1993), and the development of global capitalism (Frank 1967, Wallerstein 1982, 1993). Scant attention has been given to the effect of political development on the gendered dimension of citizenship. A number of social scientists have pointed out that theories of political development have ignored the ways in which women and men experience male-dominated political institutions differently (Aminzade 1993, Orloff 1993, Jensen 1995, Berkovitch 1999).

Some theorists have suggested that the process of political development involves both political participation and the impact of state policies on individuals (Phillips 1991, Orloff 1993, Jensen 1995, Goldberg 2001). Vilas (1995) pointed out that political development implies effectively addressing economic inequalities and articulating the demands of all socially mobilized sectors, including the improvement of women's socioeconomic status and the realization of women's rights. Jaquette and Wolchik (1998) and McDonagh (2002) argued that political development and the ideological shift from the use of ascrptive group characteristics to the liberal principles of individual equality may enable new actors, such as women to mobilize and challenge the political system and their status quo for the sake of their own well-being. Research on Africa and Latin-America has found that political development may co-opt a broader gender equality agenda (Luciak 1999, Schild 2000). In a 2008 publication, Wejnert (2008), meanwhile, questioned the perception that democratization may lead to the improvement of gender equality, arguing that the costs of democratization have been largely overlooked in terms of the its impact on the economic opportunities available to women.

In this study, gender equality is hypothesized to be positively affected by the levels of political development.

2.6 Economic Development and Women's Human Rights

It is widely acknowledged that economic development is necessary for the improvement of women's human rights. Economic development is often characterized by the process associated with rapid growth in technology and the changes in the scale of society (Kerr, Dunlop, Harbison, and Myers 2001). Dijkstra and Hanmer (2000) argued that growth in technological innovations and the knowledge-based economy as a result of economic development may, in many ways, lead to the improved status of women and women's human rights. Bell (2001), in conceptualizing post-industrial societies, suggested that gains from economic development tend to be transformed into the improvement in the well-being of people especially that of women, given the character of science and technology and the requirements of modern methods of production and distribution.

In this study, economic development is hypothesized to positively affect women's human rights.

2.7 Political Development and Women's Human Rights

One of the theoretical approaches in explaining the relationship between political development and women's human rights focuses on the changing concept of citizenship in the course of political development (Berkovitch 1999, Turner 2001, McDaniel 2002). In fact, the perception that the protection of citizenship is essential for promoting human rights is not new (Stuart 2000). More than 2,000 years ago, Aristotle affirmed that the state has the responsibility to provide its citizens with the measures of well-being including basic human rights. The new notion of citizenship suggests that all citizens have the right to a basic standard of living and health care, and economic, social, and cultural rights (Brodie 1996). Berkovitch (1999) pointed out the importance of the democratic nation-state in constituting women as a social category of citizens through legislative and organizational activities. Lamas (2001) further argued that women's rights are intimately linked to the meaning of modern citizenship regardless of the levels of economic development.

Political development is often associated with democratization, diminishing authority of religious institutions, and the widespread quest for scientific knowledge. In a new "age of reason" traditional norms are challenged by egalitarian beliefs and practices. This shift may result in the redefinition of the roles of women and their status in the family and society as well as their human rights. In a study of Afghan women, Ahmed-Ghosh (2006) found that women's rights can only be ensured through the democratic form of government where women are provided with the means to disassociate themselves from the patrilineal family structure, to negotiate their rights, and to participate fully in social, economic, and political lives. It is likely that political development may lead to an improvement in women's human rights (Pitanguy 2002).

2.8 Economic Development and Maternal-Child Care

One of the apparent gains from economic development is the changing capacity of the government to provide its people with basic social, material, and other needs, such as food, clothing, shelter, and access to basic health care, education, and social services (Estes 1984, United Nations Economic and Social Commission for Asia and the Pacific – ESCAP 1998, World Bank 2006). Estes (2007) found that rapid economic development in selected developing countries is reflected in their lower population growth rates, contraceptive prevalence, and substantial improvements in antenatal care and children immunization. Findings on maternal and child health have suggested that mortality rates have increasingly been concentrated in the poorest countries and the most marginalized sectors of society (Parker 2002, Wickrama and Lorenz 2002). Meanwhile, Smith and Ingham (2005) cautioned that the commodification of care within the economic regeneration policies that establishes care work as low-paid and insecure employment may lead to negative effect on maternal and care services.

In this study, a positive relationship between economic development and maternal-child care is hypothesized.

2.9 Political Development and Maternal-Child Care

Hagoplan (2000) identified three key features of political development, democratic governance, political representation and accountability, and organization of civil societies to differentiate them from neo-modernization theories. Political development is generally seen to promise political participation on the part of all of the sectors of social life and the advancement of social equality (Coleman 1971, Nelson 1987). As a result, social inclusion policies both nationally and locally have contributed to a better maternal and child care and the well-being of mothers and their infants (Margolis, Gay, and Humphrey 1998, Scott, Campbell, and Brown 2000).

A substantial amount of literature on epidemiological transition and public health has documented the impact of political development on the tremendous gains in women's and children's health care in many countries (Omran 1971, 1982). In this study, political development is hypothesized to positively affect maternal and child care.

The hypothesized model is presented in Figure 2.1.

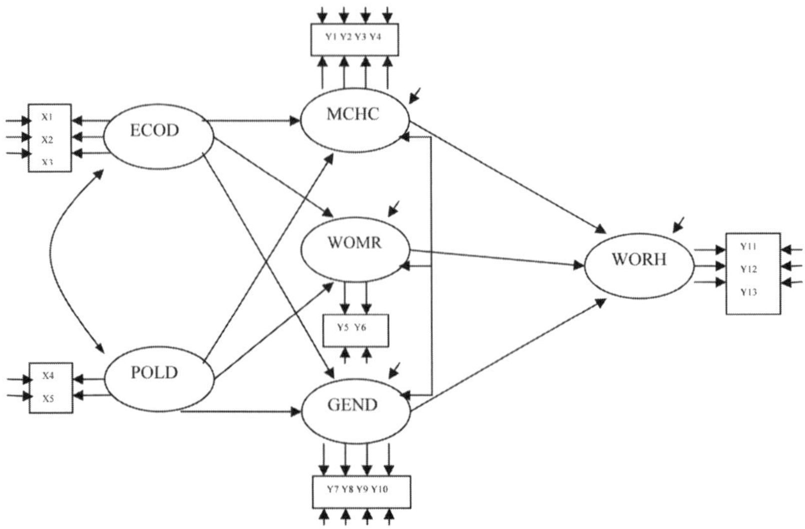

ECOD: Economic Development	X1: % population using adequate sanitation facilities X2: % population using safe water X3: % urban
POLD: Political Development	X4: political terror scale X5: Political freedom and civil liberty
MCHC: Maternal-Child Care	Y1: Skilled attendance at delivery Y2: Antenatal care coverage Y3: Children immunized against measles Y4: Contraceptive prevalence
WOMR: Women's Human Rights	Y5: Abortion right Y6: Women's economic, political, and social rights
GEND: Gender Equality	Y7: Female gross secondary enrollment Y8: Estimated female income Y9: Gender equity index Y10: Seats in parliament held by women
WORH: Women's Reproductive Health:	Y11: Infant mortality Y12: Maternal mortality Y13: Infant with low birth weight

Figure 2.1 Proposed Model

Chapter 3
Measurement of the Variables

Chapter 3 consists of three sections. The first section discusses the selection and the measurement of women's reproductive health indicators. This section includes (1) chronology of the measurement of reproductive health and (2) measurement of women's reproductive health in this study. Section two focuses on the measurement of exogenous factors: gender equality, women's human rights, maternal and child care, economic development, and political development. Descriptions of data sources are provided in the third section.

3.1 Indicators and Scales of Women's Reproductive Health

I. Chronology of the Measurement of Reproductive Health

Since the 1994 United Nations International Conference on Population and Development (ICPD) and the Fourth World Women's Conference (1995), progress has been made in terms of the data availability of reproductive health at the national and international levels. Between 1993 and 1996, the World Health Organization (WHO), together with the United Nations Children's Fund (UNICEF) and the United Nations Fund for Population Activities (UNFPA) proposed an aggregated list of 150 reproductive health indicators that are grouped in 11 program areas: (1) family planning, (2) safe motherhood (general, prenatal care, intrapartum care, essential obstetric care, postnatal care), (3) maternal nutrition, (4) newborn health and breastfeeding, (5) STD/HIV/AIDS, (6) abortion care, (7) adolescent reproductive health, (8) female genital mutilation (FGM), (9) violence against women, (10) reproductive tract cancers, and (11) infertility (WHO 1997a). Each of the 11 program areas included reflection of policy, provision, and impact. Thirty-seven variables were identified as impact variables: (1) percentage of total births to unmarried women, (2) crude birth rate, (3) total fertility rate, (4) maternal mortality ratio, (5) annual number of maternal deaths, (6) maternal mortality rate, (7) lifetime risk, (8) maternal deaths as proportion of all deaths among women of reproductive age (WRA), (9) number of deaths from maternal tetanus, (10) percentage of women with low breast-milk vitamin A, (11) proportion of all WRA anaemic (<12 g/dl) and proportion of women who are anaemic (<11 g/dl), (12) percentage of malnourished women (by body mass index), (13) percentage of newborns weighing at least 2,500g at birth, (14) percentage of low birth weight, (15) survival rate of low birth weight babies, (16) fresh/macerated stillbirth ratio, (17) neonatal mortality rate, (18) perinatal mortality rate, (19) infant mortality rate, (20) percentage of perinatal deaths contributed by stillbirth and early neonatal deaths, (21) neonatal tetanus incidence rate, (22) neonatal tetanus mortality rate, (23) <5 mortality rate (by sex), (24) estimated prevalence of syphilis and/or gonorrhea (by sex), (25) prevalence of STDs in defined target population, (26) HIV prevalence in pregnant women, (27) prevalence RPR^+ in pregnant women, (28) reported prevalence in male urethral discharge, (29) estimated prevalence of HIV among adolescents, (30) ectopic pregnancy rate, (31) annual number of (i) legal abortion (ii) estimated illegal abortions, (32) fertility rate of women 15–19 years, (33) adolescent (<20) fertility rate by year of age, (34) percentage of births to adolescent women that are wanted, (35) estimated prevalence of women who have been genitally mutilated, (36) percentage of sexually active, non-contracepting WRA (15–49) at risk of pregnancy who have not had any pregnancies in the previous five years, and (37) percentage of women 20-44 who want to become pregnant, are not using contraception and have not become pregnant during the last two years. Table 3.1 presents the 150 reproductive health indicators proposed by the World Health Organization, the United Nations Children's Fund, and the United Nations Fund for Population Activities.

A short list of reproductive health indicators was later issued by the World Health Organization (WHO). These indicators were: (1) total fertility rate, (2) contraceptive prevalence rate (CPR), (3) maternal mortality ratio (MMR), (4) percentage of women who are attended to by skilled health personnel at least once during pregnancy for reasons relating to pregnancy, (5) percentage of births attended to by skilled health personnel, (6) number of facilities with functioning basic essential obstetric care per 500,000 population, (7) number of facilities with functioning comprehensive essential obstetric care per 500,000 population, (8) perinatal mortality rate (PNMR), (9) percentage of live births of low birth weight (less than 2,500g), (10) positive syphilis serology prevalence in pregnant women (15–24), (11) percentage of women of reproductive age (15–49) screened for hemoglobin levels who are anemic, (12) percentage of obstetric and gynecological admissions owning to abortion, (13) reported prevalence of women with FGM, (14) percentage of women of reproductive age (15–49) at risk of pregnancy who report trying for two years or more, (15) reported incidence of urethritis in men, and (16) HIV prevalence in pregnant women.

Three years later, the World Health Organization (1999) recommended a list of 15 indicators to measure women's reproductive health, including: (1) total fertility rate, (2) contraceptive prevalence rate, (3) maternal mortality ratio, (4) percentage of women who are attended to by skilled health personnel (excluding trained or untrained traditional birth attendants) at least once during pregnancy for reasons relating to pregnancy, (5) percentage of births attended by skilled health personnel (excluding trained and untrained traditional birth attendants), (6) number of facilities with functioning basic essential obstetric care per 500,000 population, (7) number of facilities with functioning comprehensive essential obstetric care per 500,000 population, (8) perinatal mortality rate, (9) percentage of live births of low birth weight (less than 2,500g), (10) positive syphilis serology prevalence

Table 3.1 WHO, UNICEF, and UNFPA: List of Reproductive Health Indicators 1993–1996

Family Planning	Policy 1. Existence of a policy development plan for family planning 2. National policy for the provision of contraceptives at nominal cost or without charge 3. Legislation or policy that prohibits provision of family planning to persons (i) unmarried or (ii) below a given age Provision *measure of availability* 4. # of contraceptive methods available at primary health centers *direct output* 5. # of population within 2 hours walk from a SDP providing family planning 6. # of SDPs located within a fixed distance or travel time of a given location 7. % of family planning clients who are (i) adolescents (ii) men 8. % of women up to 6 weeks postpartum offered family planning 9. % of clients asked about their (i) reproductive intentions (ii) concerns about contraceptive methods *measure of intermediate output* 10. Proportion of WRA currently using modern contraceptive method / Contraceptive prevalence rate (by method) 11. % of WRA who want to postpone or stop childbearing who are not currently using any contraception 12. Average number of children desired Impact 13. % of total births to unmarried women 14. Crude birth rate 15. Total fertility rate
Safe Motherhood – General	Policy 16. Existence and implementation of a safe pregnancy strategic or operational plan Provision 17. Provision for (i) enquiries into maternal deaths (ii) special measures to reduce maternal mortality 18. % of maternal mortality cases reported 19. % of maternal deaths investigated 20. % of women receiving maternal services expressing satisfaction with prenatal, delivery and postnatal services Impact 21. Maternal mortality ratio 22. Annual number of maternal deaths 23. Maternal mortality rate 24. Lifetime risk 25. Maternal deaths as proportion of all deaths among WRA 26. # of deaths from maternal tetanus

Table 3.1 Continued

Safe Motherhood – Antenatal Care	Provision *Measure of direct output* 27. % of antenatal clinic clients immunized against tetanus 28. % of pregnant women attending antenatal clinic who receive iron/folate 29. % of ANC clients who have had an RPR done 30. % correct use of the home-based maternity record or the antenatal clinic record *measure of intermediate output* 31. % of women attended at least once during pregnancy by trained health personnel for reasons related to pregnancy 32. % of pregnant women attended at least once by trained health personnel 33. % of first antenatal clinic visits before quickening/1st trimester/before 16 weeks gestation 34. % of unbooked deliveries 35. % of pregnant women immunized against tetanus (TT2 or booster) 36. % of all adults knowledgeable about maternal complications of pregnancy and childbirth
Safe Motherhood – Intrapartum Care	Provision *measure of input* 37. # of "clean delivery kits" replenished from stores 38. % trained TBAs recently refreshed 39. % trained TBAs regularly supervised 40. # of institution personnel refreshed in past 12 months *measure of direct output* 41. % women who were in prolonged labor (>24 hrs) before arrival in hospital 42. % of all hospital deliveries that are births on way to hospital 43. % of labors which were induced/augmented 44. % of labors in which the partogram was used correctly 45. % of women with obstetrical complications treated within 2 hours of presentation at a health facility 46. # of referrals to a higher center *measure of intermediate output* 47. % births attended by trained health personnel (incl TBAs) 48. % births attended by trained health personnel (excl TBAs) 49. % of institutional deliveries (i) health center (ii) hospital (iii) home
Safe Motherhood – Basic and Compre-hensive Essential Obstetric Care	Provision *measure of input* 50. Availability of in-service training programs on life saving skills for midwives, nurses and paramedics *measure of direct output* 51. # health centers per 500,000 population able to provide basic essential obstetric care 52. # district hospitals per 500,000 population able to provide comprehensive essential obstetric care 53. % of women who received blood transfusion *measure of intermediate output* 54. % of women estimated to have direct obstetric complications that are seen in EOC facilities 55. % of all births that occur in facilities with EOC 56. % of district hospital deliveries considered high risk 57. Caesarean section as a proportion of all live births in the population 58. Case fatality rates for direct obstetric complications

Table 3.1 Continued

Safe Motherhood – Postnatal Care	Provision *measure of input* 59. % of service providers trained to use family planning delivery protocol for breastfeeding women 60. Contraceptive rate among nursing mothers
Maternal Nutrition	Policy 61. Existence of women's nutrition as policy priority Provision *measure of direct output* 62. % of SDPs with adequate supplies of mineral/vitamin supplements *measure of intermediate output* 63. % of pregnant clients receiving treatment for hookworm 64. % of program participants who practice key nutrition behaviors promoted by the program 65. % of households using iodized salt 66. % of women consuming vitamin A rich foods Impact 67. % of women with low breast-milk vitamin A 68. % of all WRA anemic (<12 g/dl) and proportion pregnant women who are anemic (<11 g/dl) 69. % of malnourished women (by body mass index)
Health of the Newborn and Breastfeeding	Policy 70. National breastfeeding policy and plan Provision *measure of quality care* 71. % of perinatal deaths investigated 72. % of neonatal tetanus cases delivered in institutions 73. % of neonatal tetanus cases delivered by trained TBAs *measure of availability* 74. % of service providers trained in breastfeeding counseling *measure of intermediate output* 75. % of mothers of <6/12 olds who have received support/advice about breastfeeding from community member 76. % of target audience exposed to information, education and communication messages on breastfeeding 77. % of children 20-24 months who are breastfeeding. 78. % exclusive breastfeeding up to 4 months 79. Timely complementary feeding rate – the % of infants 6-9/12 receiving complementary foods according to breastfeeding status 80. % of all adults knowledgeable about neonatal complications Impact 81. % of newborns weighing at least 2500g at birth 82. % low birth weight 83. Survival rate of low birth weight babies 84. Fresh/macerated stillbirth ratio 85. Neonatal mortality rate 86. Perinatal mortality rate 87. Infant mortality rate 88. % of perinatal deaths contributed by stillbirth and early neonatal deaths 89. Neonatal tetanus incidence rate 90. Neonatal tetanus mortality rate 91. <5 mortality rate (by sex)

Table 3.1 Continued

Prevention and Management of STD/HIV/ AIDS	Policy 92. National strategic plan to control reproductive tract infections (RTI) and STDs, including HIV/AIDS 93. Provision to protect the basic rights of HIV^+ persons with reference to employment, marriage and travel Provision *measure of input* 94. Availability of in-service training about RTIs for health providers *measure of direct output* 95. % of SDPs stocked with condoms and educational materials 96. % of SDPs offering condoms for prevention of STDs 97. % of FP/SDPs with provision of RTI/STD services 98. % of people (15–49) who can acquire a condom 99. % of SDPs offering diagnosis and treatment of (i) syphilis, (ii) gonorrhea and (iii) Chlamydia 100. # of condoms distributed 101. % of individuals presenting with STD in health facilities who are assessed and treated in an appropriate way 102. % of clients screened appropriately for RTIs before intra-uterine contraceptive device insertion 103. % of clients expressing satisfaction with RTI services *measure of intermediate output* 104. % of family planning clients who accept condoms 105. % 15–49 yrs citing two protective measures against HIV 106. % of adults practicing care-seeking behaviors that reduce STD/RTI infection 107. % of target population with unmet need for protection, i.e., % of sexually active persons who perceive selves at risk but do not report regular condom use or monogamy 108. % 15–49 yrs use of condom in last non-regular sexual intercourse 109. % of adults practicing low risk behavior for STD/HIV Impact 110. Estimated prevalence of syphilis and/or gonorrhea (by sex) 111. Prevalence of STDs in defined target population 112. HIV prevalence pregnant women 113. Prevalence RPR^+ in pregnant women 114. Reported prevalence male urethral discharge 115. Estimated prevalence of HIV among adolescents 116. Ectopic pregnancy rate
Management of Complications of Unwanted Pregnancy	Policy 117. Existence of service and administrative policy on the elements of post-abortion law Provision *measure of input* 118. Availability of in-service training on post-abortion family planning counseling for health providers *measure of direct output* 119. #, type and geographic distribution of SDPs that have commodities, equipment and transport for post abortion rate 120. % of women referred for family planning counseling after (i) legal abortion (ii) treatment for complicated abortion 121. % of women who come to a medical facility for post-abortion care who were given sufficient information to make a voluntary choice to undergo treatment and/or family planning options

Table 3.1 Continued

	122. Compliance with provisions for maintaining confidentiality 123. % of post-abortion care clients who receive counseling and referral or accept a family planning method at the time of service 124. Case fatality rates for post-abortion complications *measure of intermediate output* 125. % of obstetric and gynecological admittance/outpatients due to abortion complications 126. Total number of admissions for post-abortion complications 127. % of women with knowledge that post-abortion care is available, % that say it is acceptable, % that they would use it Impact 128. Annual number of (i) legal abortion (ii) estimated illegal abortions
Adolescent Reproductive Health	Policy 129. Existence of government policies, programs or laws favorable to adolescent reproductive health 130. Age at first marriage by sex – does a legal minimum age exist? What is the legal minimum age? Is it enforced? 131. Legislation or policy that prohibits provision of family planning to persons (i) unmarried or (ii) below a given age Provision *measure of direct output* 132. % providers who have successfully completed training on adolescent health services 133. % participants competent in communication with adolescents in reproductive health issues 134. # of SDPs serving adolescents that are located within a fixed distance or travel time of a given location *measure of intermediate output* 135. Total # of contacts with adolescents 136. % of family planning clients who are (i) adolescents (ii) men. 137. % adolescents who know of at least one source of information and/or services for sexual and reproductive health 138. Adolescent's knowledge of reproductive health (composite index) 139. % adolescents who used protection at first/most recent sexual intercourse 140. Adolescent contraceptive user and/or non-user characteristics
	Impact 141. Fertility rate of women 15–19 years 142. Adolescent (<20) fertility rate by year of age 143. % of births to adolescent women that are wanted
Female Genital Mutilation	Policy 144. Implementation of policy measures to eliminate (i) female genital mutilation (ii) prenatal sex selection Impact 145. Estimated prevalence of women who have been genitally mutilated
Violence against Women	Impact 146. Sex ratio of births (M:F>107–100 ? prenatal sex selection)

Table 3.1 Concluded

Screening and Treatment of Cancers of the Reproductive Tract	Provision *measure of availability* 147. % of SDPs (i) offering PAP testing *measure of intermediate output* 148. % of women aged 35–59 examined at least once for cancer of the cervix
Infertility	Impact 149. % of sexually active, non-contracepting WRA (15–49) at risk of pregnancy who have not had any pregnancies in the previous 5 years 150. % of women 20–44 who want to become pregnant, are not using contraception and have not become pregnant during the last 2 years

Source: World Health Organization (WHO). 1997a. *Monitoring Reproductive Health: Selecting a Short List of National and Global Indicators*. Geneva: WHO.

in pregnant women (15–24), (11) percentage of women of reproductive age (15–49) screened for hemoglobin levels who are anemic, (12) percentage of obstetric and gynecological admissions owning to abortion, (13) reported prevalence of women with FGM, (14) percentage of women of reproductive age (15–49) who report trying for a pregnancy for two years or more, and (15) reported incidence of urethritis in men (15–49). Two more indicators were later added to the list: (1) HIV prevalence in pregnant women and (2) knowledge of HIV-related prevention practices. All of above three lists of indicators recommended by the World Health Organization, the United Nations Children's Fund and the United Nations Fund for Population Activities identified infant and maternal health as women's reproductive health indicators.

At the same time, the United States Agency for International Development (USAID 1999) put together a three-level hierarchy of indicators that contained 29 variables. Higher-level indicators were considered to reflect trends in reproductive health; the second-level indicators were defined as tracking people-level impact in terms of the use of services or other behavior; and the third-level indicators were defined as monitoring progress in improving access to family planning and reproductive health services. Table 3.2 presents the reproductive health indicators proposed by the US Agency for International Development.

The World Health Organization (WHO 1999, 2001) further recommended that reproductive health indicators include those variables that can be used to monitor changes in reproductive health status and service utilization over time and across regions, and can facilitate the achievement of specific goals and objectives. The World Health Organization (WHO 2002) later suggested adding the health of the newborn, promotion of positive sexual health, and violence against women to the list. In addition, Population Action International (PAI 2001) used a composite index of reproductive health risks to measure women's reproductive health. The index consisted of total fertility rate, contraception prevalence rate, policies towards abortion, proportion of pregnant women with anaemia, prenatal care, delivery assistance, HIV in women, infertility in women, and maternal mortality rates.

Table 3.2 Hierarchy of Reproductive Health Indicators

Higher-level indicators	Second-level indicators	Third-level indicators
Total fertility rate	1. Family planning:	Access to services
HIV/STI prevalence or incidence	Contraceptive prevalence rate	Quality of services
Under-five mortality rate	Couple-years of protection	Demand (knowledge, attitudes, or practices)
Nutritional status	2. Child survival:	Sustainability (establishment of sustainable family planning and health programs and services)
Infant mortality	Immunization coverage	
Prevalence of vitamin A deficiency	Oral rehydration therapy use rate	
Maternal mortality ratio	Treatment of acute respiratory infections	
	Treatment of fever (presumptive malaria)	
	Infant feeding practices	
	Exclusive breastfeeding	
	Complementary feeding	
	Vitamin A supplementation	
	3. Mental health:	
	Births attended by medical personnel	
	Use of prenatal services	
	4. HIV/STI prevention:	
	Reported condom use with non-regular partner	
	Reported condom use with regular partner	
	Reported non-regular sexual partners	
	Treatment of STIs	
	5. Infectious diseases:	
	Use of insecticide-treated bed nets	
	Prevention of malaria among pregnant women	

Source: United States Agency for International Development (USAID). 1999.

The United Nations Fund for Population Activities (UNFPA 2001), meanwhile, proposed six variables to measure reproductive health: (1) infant mortality, (2) life expectancy, (3) maternal mortality rate, (4) births per 1,000 women aged 15–19, (5) contraceptive prevalence, and (6) HIV prevalence rate.

In 2003, the Population Reference Bureau (PRB) and the United Nations Fund for Population Activities (UNFPA) put together a list of reproductive health indicators, including maternal mortality per 100,000 live births, infant mortality per 1,000 live births, under age 5 mortality rate, and HIV/AIDS prevalence for adolescents (aged 15–24). The following year, the United Nations Fund for Population Activities (UNFPA) recommended 17 reproductive health indicators: (1) total number of children a woman would have by the end of her reproductive period, (2) percentage of women of reproductive age (15–49) who are using (or whose partner is using) a contraceptive method at a particular point in time, (3) number of maternal deaths per 100,000 live births, (4) percentage of women who are attended to by skilled health personnel (excluding trained or untrained traditional birth attendants) at least once during pregnancy for reasons relating to pregnancy, (5) percentage of births attended to by skilled health personnel (excluding trained and untrained traditional birth attendants), (6) number of facilities with functioning basic essential obstetric care per 500,000 population*,[1] (7) number of facilities with functioning comprehensive essential obstetric care per 500,000 population*, (8) number of perinatal deaths per 1,000 total births*, (9) percentage of live births that weigh less than 2500g, (10) percentage of pregnant women aged 15 to 24 attending antenatal care clinics, whose blood has been screened for syphilis, with positive serology for syphilis*, (11) percentage of women of reproductive age (15–49) screened for hemoglobin levels with levels below 110g/1 for pregnant women, and below 120g/1 for non-pregnant women*, (12) percentage of all cases admitted to service delivery points, providing in-patient obstetric and gynecological services, which are due to abortion (spontaneous and induced, but excluding planned termination of pregnancy)*, (13) percentage of women interviewed in a community survey, reporting themselves to have undergone FGM*, (14) percentage of women of reproductive age (15–49) at risk of pregnancy (not pregnant, sexually active, non-contracepting and non-lactating) who report trying for a pregnancy for two years or more*, (15) percentage of men aged 15–49 interviewed in a community survey reporting episodes of urethritis in the last 12 months*, (16) percentage of pregnant women aged 15–24 attending antenatal clinics, whose blood has been screened for HIV and who are seropositive for HIV*, and (17) percentage of all respondents who correctly identify all three major ways of preventing the sexually transmission of HIV and who reject three major misconceptions about HIV transmission or prevention*.

Dixon-Mueller and Germain (2006) later proposed adding the following outcome variables to measure women's reproductive health: (1) proportion of

1 "*" indicates that data are either not available or have 30 percent or more missing cases.

demand for family planning satisfied, (2) availability of emergency obstetric care, (3) proportion of all births that are mistimed or unwanted, and (4) proportion of all abortions that are unsafe. In 2006, the Centers for Disease Control and Prevention (CDC) suggested 16 reproductive health indicators in six different categories: (1) fetal and infant mortality, (2) infant health, (3) pregnancy outcomes, (4) maternal risks, (5) teen risks, and (6) maternal interventions. Table 3.3 presents the 16 variables proposed by the Centers for Disease Control and Prevention.

Table 3.4 presents the chronology of reproductive health indicators recommended by the World Health Organization (WHO), the United Nations Children's Fund (UNICEF), the United Nations Fund for Populations Activities (UNFPA), the

Table 3.3 CDC Reproductive Health Indicators

Fetal and Infant Mortality	Infant Health	Pregnancy Outcomes	Maternal Risks	Teen Risks	Maternal Interventions
Infant mortality rate (infant deaths per 1,000 live births)	Low birth weight rate (number of live born infants with a birth weight less than 2,500 grams per 100 live births)	Fertility rate (number of women who had a live born infant per 1,000 women)	Smoking percent (number of women who had a live birth and smoked tobacco at any time during her pregnancy per 100 women who had a live birth)	Educational attainment percent (number of teen women who had a live birth and who were more than two years older than expected for grade level per 100 teen women who had a live birth)	1st trimester care – prenatal care began in the 1st trimester of pregnancy percent (number of women who had a live born infant who began their prenatal care in the 1st trimester of pregnancy per 100 women who had a live birth)
Neonatal mortality rate (deaths of infants less than 28 days old per 1,000 live births	Very low birth weight rate (number of live born infants with a birth weight less than 1,500 grams per 100 live births)	Fetal loss rate (number of women who had a dead born infant per 100,000 women)	Unmarried percent (number of unmarried women who had a live birth per 100 women who had a live birth)	Late/no care – prenatal care began in the 3rd trimester or no prenatal care percent (number of teen women who had a live birth and received no prenatal care or prenatal care was begun in the 3rd trimester per 100 teen women who had a live birth)	

Table 3.3 Continued

Postneonatal mortality rate (death of infants age 28 days to 1 year per 1,000 live births)	Preterm delivery rate (number of live born infants with a gestational age at delivery of less that 37 weeks per 100 live births)		Educational attainment percent (number of women who had a live birth and had attained less than a high school education at the time of delivery per 100 women who had a live birth)		
Perinatal mortality rate (perinatal deaths per 1,000 live births)			Multiple gestation percent (number of women who had a live birth and gestation with two or more fetuses per 100 women who had a live birth)		

Source: Centers for Diseases Control and Prevention (CDC). 2006a. *Reproductive Health Indicators*.

United States Agency for International Development (USAID), Centers for Diseases Control and Prevention (CDC), Population Action International (PAI), and Dixon-Mueller and Germain.

In the face of the multiplicity of reproductive health indicators, ambiguity and the lack of the validation of its measurement still exist. Harald Hansluwka, as early as 1985, reminded us that there are four difficulties in selecting health indicators: the vagueness of the concept, the value judgment of the definer (individual, or physician, or family, etc.), the multidimensionality of the phenomenon, and the impossibility of meaningful operationalization. Hansluwka (1985) suggested that one way to overcome the problems is to adopt simplifying strategies to deal with some of these problems.

In selecting and formulating indicators, social scientists and policy makers have since developed criteria to measure reproductive health. For example, Bertrand and Tsui (1995) proposed a typology of four types of indicators to measure reproductive health, namely input, process, output, and outcome indicators. Input indicators refer

Table 3.4 Chronology of Reproductive Health Indicators

Organization	Year	Types of Indicators
World Health Organization (WHO), United Nations Children's Fund (UNICEF), United Nations Fund for Population Activities (UNFPA)	1993–1996	150 indicators in 11 program areas: (1) family planning, (2) safe motherhood, (3) maternal nutrition, (4) newborn health and breastfeeding, (5) STD/HIV/AIDS, (6) abortion care, (7) adolescent reproductive health, (8) female genital mutilation (FGM), (9) violence against women, (10) reproductive tract cancers, and (11) infertility. (see Table 3.1 for the 150 indicators)
World Health Organization (WHO)	1993–1996	Short list of indicators, including (1) infant mortality, (2) contraceptive prevalence, (3) maternal mortality, (4) % women attended to by skilled health personnel, (5) % births attended to by skilled health personnel, (6) number of facilities with functioning basic essential obstetric care per 500,000 population, (7) number of facilities with functioning comprehensive essential obstetric care per 500,000 population, (8) perinatal mortality, (9) % live births of low birth weight, (10) positive syphilis serology prevalence in pregnant women (15–24), (11) % women of reproductive age screened for hemoglobin levels who are anemic, (12) % obstetric and gynecological admissions owning to abortion, (13) reported prevalence of women with FGM, (14) % women of reproductive age at risk of pregnancy who report trying for two years or more, (15) reported incidence of urethritis in men, and (16) HIV prevalence in pregnant women.
World Health Organization (WHO)	1999	17 indicators including (1) total fertility rate, (2) contraceptive prevalence, (3) maternal mortality, (4) % women attended to by skilled health personnel at least once during pregnancy, (5) % births attended by skilled health personnel, (6) number of facilities with functioning basic essential obstetric care per 500,000 population, (7) number of facilities with functioning comprehensive essential obstetric care per 500,000 population, (8) perinatal mortality, (9) % live births of low birth weight, (10) positive syphilis serology prevalence in pregnant women (15–24), (11) % women of reproductive age screened for hemoglobin levels who are anemic, (12) % obstetric and gynecological admissions owning to abortion, (13) reported prevalence of women with FGM, (14) % women of reproductive age who report trying for a pregnancy for two years or more, (15) reported incidence of urethritis in men, (16) HIV prevalence in pregnant women, and (17) knowledge of HIV-related prevention practices.
United States Agency for International Development (USAID)	1999	Three-level hierarchy of indicators including 29 variables. (see Table 3.2)
Population Action International (PAI)	2001	Composite index of reproductive health risks, including (1) total fertility rate, (2) contraception prevalence, (3) policies towards abortion, (4) % pregnant women with anaemia, (5) prenatal care, (6) delivery assistance, (7) HIV in women, (8) infertility in women, and (9) maternal mortality.

Table 3.4 Continued

United Nations Fund for Population Activities (UNFPA)	2001	Six reproductive health indicators including: (1) infant mortality, (2) life expectancy, (3) maternal mortality, (4) births per 1,000 women aged 15–19, (5) contraceptive prevalence, and (6) HIV prevalence.
World Health Organization (WHO)	2001, 2002	Suggested adding three more variables: (1) health of the newborn, (2) promotion of positive sexual health, and (3) violence against women.
United Nations Fund for Population Activities (UNFPA), Population Reference Bureau (PRB)	2003	Social-economic health and adolescent productive health indicators, including (1) maternal mortality per 100,000 live births, (2) infant mortality per 1,000 live births, (3) under age 5 mortality rate, and (4) HIV/AIDS prevalence for adolescents (aged 15–24).
United Nations Fund for Population Activities (UNFPA)	2004	17 indicators including (1) number of children a woman would have by the end of her reproductive period, (2) % women of reproductive age who are using (or whose partner is using) a contraceptive method at a particular point in time, (3) number of maternal deaths per 100,000 live births, (4) % women who are attended to by skilled health personnel, (5) % births attended to by skilled health personnel, (6) number of facilities with functioning basic essential obstetric care per 500,000 population, (7) number of facilities with comprehensive essential obstetric care per 500,000 population, (8) number of perinatal deaths per 1,000 total births, (9) % live births that weigh less than 2500g, (10) % pregnant women aged 15 to 24 attending antenatal care clinics whose blood has been screened for syphilis, with positive serology for syphilis, (11) % women of reproductive age screened for hemoglobin levels, (12) % all cases admitted to service delivery points, providing in-patient obstetric and gynecological services, which are due to abortion, (13) % women interviewed in a community survey, reporting themselves to have undergone FGM, (14) % women of reproductive age at risk of pregnancy who report trying for a pregnancy for two years or more, (15) % men aged 15–49 interviewed in a community survey reporting episodes of urethritis in the last 12 months, (16) % pregnant women aged 15–24 attending antenatal clinics, whose blood has been screened for HIV and who are seropositive for HIV, and (17) % all respondents who correctly identify all three major ways of preventing the sexually transmission of HIV and who reject three major misconceptions about HIV transmission or prevention.
Germain and Dixon-Mueller	2006	Suggested adding four outcome variables: (1) % demand for family planning satisfied, (2) availability of emergency obstetric care, (3) % all births that are mistimed or unwanted, and (4) % all abortions that are unsafe.
Centers for Disease Control and Prevention (CDC)	2006	16 indicators in six categories: (1) fetal and infant mortality, (2) infant health, (3) pregnancy outcomes, (4) maternal risks, (5) teen risks, and (6) maternal interventions. (see Table 3.3 for the 16 variables)

to the resources that are invested in a program, such as financial, technological, and human resources. Process indicators measure the activities carried out to achieve program objectives. Output indicators measure the results achieved at the program level. Outcome indicators refer to the changes at the program or population level, as well as the impact or the changes in fertility, morbidity, or mortality that can be directly attributed to the program. The World Health Organization (WHO 1997b), in line with the United Nations Development Programme (UNDP), the United Nations Fund for Population Activities (UNFPA), and the World Bank, recommended six criteria for selecting reproductive health indicators: (1) Is the indicator ethical? An indicator requires data which are ethical to collect, process, and present in terms of the rights of the individual to confidentiality, freedom of choice in supplying the data, and informed consent regarding the nature and implications of the required data. (2) Is the indicator useful? An indicator must be able to act as a "marker of progress" toward improved reproductive health status, either as a direct or proxy measure of impact or as a measure of progress toward specified progress goals. (3) Is the indicator valid and scientifically robust? An indicator must be a valid, specific, sensitive, and reliable reflection of that which it purports to measure. (4) Is the indicator representative? An indicator must adequately encompass all of the issues or population groups it is expected to cover. (5) Is the indicator understandable? An indicator must be simple to define and its value must be easy to interpret in terms of reproductive health status. (6) Is the data for the indicator accessible? The data required for an indicator should be available or relatively easy to acquire by feasible data collection methods that have been validated in field trials.

The World Health Organization (WHO 2001) further specified four principles to ensure the scale properties in addition to the face validity of the selected items. First, the scale items should be robust, which is often achieved by selecting scale items that are specific and useful in identifying changes easily over time. Second, each item should be clearly identified and defined. Third, items that are conceptually related should be identified as groups or categories. Identification of sub-dimensions within the scale is desirable. Finally, item selections are limited by data availability. As more and more relevant indicators become available, the number of scale items may be expanded. Sadana (2002), in addition, recommended three criteria for developing instruments to measure reproductive health: (1) the range of domains and subsequent indicators tested are linked to the ICPD definition, (2) the full range of health status (spanning gynecological, obstetric, contraceptive morbidity and related events) may be measured with acceptable levels of reliability and validity, and (3) measurements allow for the comparison and interpretation of reproductive health within and across populations.

Malhotra, Schuler, and Boender (2002), meanwhile, proposed two basic principles, first, to reply on a consistent conceptual framework and second, to allow flexibility in the specific indicators used to define the key components. That is, when taking into consideration data availability, developing valid indicators involves not only conceptual structure, (each item should be clearly identified and conceptually related) but also the statistical properties of the variables selected for inclusion.

Given the large array of reproductive health indicators and the criteria used for selecting reproductive health indicators, social scientists and some policy makers have acknowledged the need to address the methodological issues related to the measurement of reproductive health. As Jacobson (2000) pointed out, the methodological issues relating to the measurement of reproductive health have not been adequately addressed and; one of the obstacles that has hindered the progress of women's reproductive health conditions is the lack of conceptual and operational meanings of reproductive health and related key concepts. Sen, George, and Ostlin (2002) argued for a quantitative research methodology with variables properly defined and adequately measured.

II. Measurement of Women's Reproductive Health

Early health status assessments relied heavily on statistical data about morbidity and mortality due mostly to infectious diseases. As a result of social, technological, and medical advancement, basic survival became less problematic and people began to see health as much more than the absence of diseases and disorder, or sufferings from any designated undesirable conditions. As early as 1946, the World Health Organization (WHO) declared in its constitution that "Health is a state of complete physical, mental and social well-being and not merely the absence of disease or infirmity." (WHO 1946: Chapter 1).

The first global agenda for women's reproductive health was agreed upon at the 1994 United Nations International Conference on Population and Development (ICDP) and reaffirmed at the Fourth World Women's Conference held one year later in Beijing, China. The Platform of Action adopted at the ICDP defined reproductive health as:

> ... a state of complete physical, mental, and social well-being and not merely the absence of diseases or infirmity, in all matters relating to the reproductive system and to its functions and processes. Reproductive health therefore implies that people are able to have a satisfying and safe sex life and that they have capability to reproduce and the freedom to decide if, when, and how often to do so. Implicit in this last condition are the right of men and women to be informed and to have access to safe, effective, affordable and acceptable methods of family planning of their choice, as well as other methods of their choice for regulation of fertility which are not against the law, and the right of access to appropriate health-care services that will enable women to go safely through pregnancy and childbirth and provide couples with the best chance of having a healthy infant. (Quoted from: 96, C. Women and Health, Beijing Declaration and Platform for Action, Fourth World Conference on Women, 15 September 1995. A/CONF. 177/20, 1995 and A/CONF.177/20/Add.1, 1995)

This definition is considered to have marked a paradigm shift away from a narrow and biomedical approach. It has been frequently used as an operational basis for interventions and programs implemented by the international community and governments to monitor progress. Castle, Traore, and Cisse (2002), however, cautioned against the definition put forward by the Cairo and Beijing Conferences, arguing that the definition may not accurately reflect the attributes emerging from recent cross-country research, although this definition comprises a substantial step forward in viewing reproductive health as a well-being.

There has been no international consensus thus far in terms of a methodologically valid measure of women's reproductive health (WORH), although numerous indicators have been developed (International Planned Parenthood Federation – IPPF 2002). Recently, social scientists and medical practitioners acknowledged the importance of maternal and child health outcomes as critical measures of women's reproductive health. Beginning around 1985, Rosenfield and Maine looked at what is called the maternal-child health field (MCH). In a 1993 publication in the *Health Transition Review*, Zuray, Khattab, Younis, El-Mouelhy, and Fadle found that child survival and safe motherhood are important indicators of women's reproductive health in developing countries. Bennett (1997) suggested that women's health and reproductive health issues be incorporated fully into the field of MCH. In Bennette's analysis of women's health, three variables were used, low birth weight, infant mortality, and severe maternal complications. Pachauri (1999) further argued that reproductive health be situated in maternal and infant survival and well-being.

For this study, the selection of the scale items to measure women's reproductive health is guided by the principles set forth by Bollen (1990)[2], the World Health Organization (WHO 2001), and Malhortra, Schuler, and Boender (2002) that, in developing valid reproductive health indicators, we should keep in mind not only the conceptual structure but also the statistical properties of the variables selected for inclusion while taking into consideration data availability (Malhortra, Schuler, and Boender 2002). The selection of the scale items to measure women's reproductive health in this study is also guided by the conceptual and operational characterization of the variables as well as the operational model proposed by Rosenfield and Maine (1985), Zuray, Khattab, Younis, El-Mouelhy, and Fadle (1993), Bennette (1997), and Claeson, Bos, Mawji, and Pathmanathan (2000) to incorporate women's health and reproductive health issues in MCH.

In this study, the women's reproductive health indicators are expressed in rates, ratios, and proportions. Three variables are used to measure women's reproductive health: (1) infant mortality rate (per 1,000 live births), (2) maternal mortality

2 Bollen (1990) suggested six standards in his study on the measurement of political democracy: (1) provide a theoretical definition, (2) identify major dimensions, (3) measure each dimension with several indicators, (4) explain how indicators were created and how to replicate them, (5) specify the relations between each dimension and the indicator, and (6) report estimate of reliability and validity.

ratio (100,000 live births),[3] and (3) percentage of infants with low birth weight (infants who weigh less than 2,500 grams). All reproductive health variables are continuous variables.

In the next section, I will discuss the selection of the measurement scales of the exogenous factors.

3.2 Indicators of Exogenous Variables

The exogenous dimensions of this study include maternal-child care (MCHC), gender equality (GEND), women's rights (WOMR), economic development (ECOD), and political development (POLD).

I. Maternal-Child Care

The World Health Organization (World Health Organization 2006 a, b), in collaboration with the United States Agency for International Development (USAID 2006), suggested five areas for assessing maternal and child care: (1) pre-conception/inter-conception care, (2) antenatal care, (3) labor and delivery, (4) postpartum care, and (5) newborn care. In a study of maternal and child care programs in Eritrea, Gottlieb and Lindmark (2002) recommended six indicators to evaluate maternal and child health care programs: (1) proportion of women who are attended to by trained staff at least once during pregnancy, (2) proportion of births that are attended to by trained staff, (3) number of health centers providing EOC (essential obstetric care) per 500,000 population, (4) proportion of complicated cases managed at EOC facilities, (5) C-sections as a proportion of all births in the population, and (6) percentage of population within one hour travel time to EOC facility. The World Health Organization (WHO 2009) and United Nations Children's Fund (UNICEF 2009) suggested a number of measures pertaining to maternal and child health care, including adequate antenatal care, postnatal care, skilled assistance at delivery, and immunization.

In this study, four variables are used to measure maternal and child care: (1) percentage of deliveries who are attended to by skilled attendants (skilled),[4] (2)

---

3 Due to systematic underreporting and misreporting of maternal deaths in some developing countries, the reliability of current available data sources vary; and accurate monitoring of progress depends on better systems of surveillance and registration (United Nations 2009).

4 The World Health Organization (WHO 2005) defined skilled attendance as "a health provider who has at least the minimum knowledge and skills to manage normal childbirth and provide basic (first line) emergency obstetric care. A skilled attendant should be able to perform the following functions: (1) safely conduct a normal delivery using aseptic technique, (2) active management of the third stage of labor, (3) provide immediate care of the newborn including resuscitation, (4) manage most postpartum hemorrhage through

percentage of pregnant women aged 15–49 who are attended to by skilled health personnel at least once during pregnancy (antenatal), (3) percentage of one-year old children who are immunized against measles (measles), and (4) percentage of women aged 15–49 currently using contraception (contraception). All maternal-child care variables are continuous variables.

II. Gender Equality

Gender equality as a development goal has been recognized in the policy statements put forth at several international conferences, for instance, the Cairo Program of Action (ICPD 1994), the Beijing Platform for Action (United Nations 1995), and the Millennium Declaration (United Nations 2000a, b). The literature pertaining to the concept shows that a variety of terms has been used to describe the gender-related power discrepancies and women's inferior social and economic status in society. One of the earliest studies by Acharya (1979, 1981) used a more general term "women's status" to refer to the levels of women's control over economic resources and life options. Other terms that have been used include female (women's) power, female autonomy, gender stratification (or discrimination), and women's empowerment. A 2001 World Bank report used the term gender equality to refer to the characteristics and the processes with regard to women's social, economic, and political status at the aggregate level.

Chafetz (1991) considered gender equality encompassing (1) a division of labor between women and men and (2) power at the macro level. Mason (1995) defined gender equality as "a gender system's expectations" that "prescribe a division of labor and responsibilities between women and men and grant different rights and obligations to them." (p. 1). Rudd (2000) saw gender equality as a "sorting mechanism in an increasingly stratified society" that affects gender relations by increasing the social value of paid work relative to family activities (p. 518). According to Rudd, women confront two types of losses as a result. The first is the discrimination in the labor market that pushes women out of paid employment and back into the home and forces them to depend on men economically. The second is a form of social devaluation of family work. Taylor-Gooby (1991) and Lewis (2000) pointed out the consequences of devaluing unpaid family work which is primarily done by women. First, women's continued responsibility for the bulk of unpaid domestic labor simultaneously limits their access to the labor market. Second, while a greater number of women have entered the labor force, their

---

use of parenteral oxytocics and abdominal massage, (5) mutually remove the placenta, (6) manage eclampsia through provision of parenteral antihypertensives, (7) recognize and manage postpartum infection through use of parenteral antibiotics, (8) perform assisted vaginal delivery through use of a vacuum extractor, (9) manage incomplete abortions with manual vacuum aspiration, and (10) know how to refer women to the next level of care and stabilize them for their journey (United Nations Children's Fund, World Health Organization, and United Nations Fund for Population Activities 1997).

pay status remains lower than that of men. The labor market is organized on the assumption that women's wages are secondary to a male-breadwinning wage. The economic logic generated by unequal labor market rewards tends to encourage a traditional domestic division of labor mostly done by women. Women's economic dependency on men is likely to result in women's carrying out unpaid domestic work, thus lessening the degree of autonomy (Hobson 1994, Lewis 2000). Therefore, different economic rewards from domestic work and the labor market participation can translate into differences in power within the family and in the society. Dunn, Almquist, and Chafetz (1993) considered it an extremely difficult task that remains to be accomplished if a comprehensive operational definition of gender equality is to be developed.

Given the intricacy in conceptualizing gender equality, Penna and Campbell (1998) and Mason and Smith (2003) warned of the complexity in developing relevant indicators to measure the concept especially in cross country studies. Ackerly (1995) argued that gender equality is a process as opposed to a condition or a state of being, and therefore, can only be measured by proxies. Mason (1986), citing the work by Whyte (1978), argued that gender equality is empirically and conceptually a multidimensional phenomenon, meaning that women who are powerless in one area may not be necessarily powerless in other areas in comparison to their male counterparts. For example, women may be given considerable power in making financial decisions within the family, and simultaneously derived of the freedom to run for political offices and seek employment outside home. Mason (1986) and Mason and Smith (2003) further suggested that gender equality should be a property of the social system and studied at the aggregate rather than individual level. Therefore, macro-dimensional conceptualizations as well as operational and measurement schemes of the concept are of primary importance.

In developing indicators of gender equality, Mason (1986) warned against some problems. One of the problems concerns conceptual ambiguity and the failure to clearly define the concept. The other problem is related to the selection of indicators that may imply conflicting connotations and Mason called it "the problem of context dependency." (p. 294). For example, one of the most frequently used indicators, women's labor force participation, may enhance gender equality in some societies but not necessarily in some other societies. In sub-Saharan Africa, for example, women's overall representation in the labor force is relatively high, about 55 percent of working-age women in the region are employed. However, close to two thirds of all employed women have vulnerable jobs and only 23 percent of these women are employed in industry and 21 percent are working in the service sector (United Nations 2009).

Several efforts have been made in recent years to construct measures of gender equality. The United Nations Development Program (UNDP 1990, 1995) identified gender-related development index (GDI) as a measure of gender equality,[5] and

5 GDI is a derivative of the human development index (HDI). It is calculated from the differences between men and women with regard to life expectancy, education, and income.

subsequently GEM (gender empowerment measure), and GEI (gender equality index). Morgan (2001), however, considered none of the three measures alone as crude measures of gender equality because they cannot measure "the degree to which social pressures obstruct or prevent a women's exercise of her legal rights." (p. 2). Thus far, a rigorous method for measuring and tracking changes in gender equality has not been adequately developed (Sen 1994, Malhotra, Schuler, and Boender 2002); and there is no single measure of gender equality (Riley 1997, Wang 2004).

Mason (1998) and Morgan (2001) suggested that women's economic decision making power in the family should be a measure of gender equality. Kritz, Makinwa-Adebusoye, and Gurak (2000) put forward an index of eight indicators in their research of the four communities in Nigeria, including percentages of wives in modern work and percentages of wives who have control over the use of income. Kishor (2000) further suggested that levels of education and employment should be used as proxy variables. The empirical work by Blood and Wolfe (1960) was among the first to consider money as a critical variable that may affect gender relations. Safilios-Rothschild (1982) considered women's economic independence and having a stable and adequate financial base to be a critical measure of gender equality. Malhotra, Schuler, and Boender (2002) included women's control over income, women's representation in high paying jobs, and women's literacy and access to a broad range of educational options as potential indicators of gender equality.[6] Based on the conceptual framework and data availability, gender equality in this study is measured by the following four variables: (1) female gross secondary enrollment, (enroll), (2) estimated female earned income (income),[7] (3) gender equity index (gei),[8] and (4) percentage of seats in parliament held by women (seats). All gender equality indicators are continuous variables.

---

6 Fathalla (1993) pointed out three questionable consequences when female education alone is used to measure gender equality. First, it masks the power dimension and multifaceted nature of gender relations although education may reduce some power imbalance. Second, it downplays other aspects of gender relations; and third, emphasis on formal education alone ignores state responsibilities to provide social services and other basic needs. Cross-national data on women's political participation, such as the percentage served in parliament are highly skewed. Women's share of labor force participation may not adequately reveal the nature of gender equality and the full range of women's possible options. First, high work force participation may not imply increasing empowerment. Second, it fails to reflect women's work at home or in the informal sectors (United Nations Fund for Population Activites 2000).

7 Data for female earned income are crude estimates (United Nations Development Programme 2008).

8 Gender equality index (gei) includes three dimensions: economic activity, empowerment, and education with 0 indicating the lowest level and 100 the highest level of gender equity.

III. Women's Human Rights

The idea of human rights originated from the early philosophical, sociological, and legal propositions of natural law and natural rights that individuals are entitled to certain immutable rights (Pillai and Wang 1999). The development of socialism in the 19th century expanded the concept of individual rights as natural rights to social entitlement. As described in The Universal Declaration of Human Rights (1948), these rights include the right to an adequate standard of living, the right to education, the right to work, the right to just and favorable conditions of work, and the right to protection against unemployment. It was not until the 1920s that the international community began to address the rights issues especially concerning women (Appendix D. Women's Human Rights and Reproductive Rights). Hellsten (2000) acknowledged the challenges in developing a globally acceptable set of variables of women's human rights primarily due to the debate between ethical universalism and cultural relativism.

Cook and Bernard (2003) suggested that women's human rights include equal citizenship with men and women's choices for reproductive self determination. Walsh, Mollmann and Heimburger (2008) further reaffirmed that access to safe and legal abortion is a central human right issue for women in spite of the fact that most of the human right treaties do not refer directly to abortion right.

In this study, two variables are used to measure women's human rights: (1) abortion right (abortion) and (2) women's economic, political, and social rights (EPS-rights). Abortion right is divided into nine categories based on the legal status of abortion and the conditions that abortion is permitted: (1) illegal with no exceptions, (2) only when a pregnancy threatens a woman's life, (3) under life-threatening circumstances on the grounds of "necessity", (4) in case of fetal impairment, (5) to preserve women's physical health, (6) to preserve women's mental health, (7) in case of rape and/or incest, (8) on socio-economic grounds, and (9) without restriction as to reason. A country is coded 0 if abortion is illegal. Each of the other categories is coded 1. The scale of the abortion right variable ranges from 0 to 8.

The women's human rights variable is a composite measure of women's political rights, economic rights, and social rights (Cingranelli and Richards 2008). Women's political rights include the right to vote, the right to run for political office, the right to hold elected and appointed government positions, the right to join political parties, and the right to petition government officials. A score of 0 indicates that none of women's political rights is guaranteed by law. A score of 1 indicates that women's political rights are guaranteed in law, but that there are significant limitations in practice and that women hold less than 5 percent of the seats in the national legislature and in other high-ranking government positions. A score of 2 indicates that women's political rights are guaranteed in law, but that these rights are still moderately prohibited in practice and that women hold 5 percent but less than 30 percent of the seats in the national legislature and/or in other high-ranking government positions. A score of 3 indicates that women's political rights are guaranteed in law and in practice, and that women hold more than 30 percent of the seats in the national legislature and/or in other high-ranking government positions (Cingranelli and Richards 2008).

Women's economic rights consist of ten internationally recognized rights: (1) equal pay for equal work, (2) free choice of profession or employment without the need to obtain a consent from the husband or male relative, (3) the right to gainful employment without the need to obtain a consent from the husband or male relative, (4) equality in hiring and promotion practices, (5) job security (such as, maternal leave, unemployment benefits, no arbitrary firing or layoffs, etc.), (6) non-discrimination by employers, (7) the right to be free from sexual harassment in the workplace, (8) the right to work at night, (9) the right to work in occupations classified as dangerous, and (10) the right to work in the military and the police force. A score of 0 indicates that there are no economic rights for women in law and that systematic discrimination against women may have been built into law. A score of 1 indicates that women have some economic rights under law, but that these rights are not effectively enforced. A score of 2 indicates that women have some economic rights under law and that the government effectively enforces these rights in practice while still allowing a low level of discrimination against women in economic matters. A score of 3 indicates that all or nearly all of women's economic rights are guaranteed by law and that the government fully and vigorously enforces these laws in practice (Cingranelli and Richards 2008).

Twelve rights categories are specified to measure women's social rights: (1) the right to equal inheritance, (2) the right to enter into marriage on the basis of equality with men, (3) the right to travel abroad, (4) the right to obtain passport, (5) the right to confer citizenship to children or a husband, (6) the right to initiate a divorce, (7) the right to own, acquire, manage, and retain property brought into marriage, (8) the right to participate in social, cultural, and community activities, (9) the right to an education, (10) the freedom to choose a residence/domicile, (11) the freedom from female genital mutilation (FGM) of children and of adults without their consent, and (12) the freedom from forced sterilization. A score of 0 is assigned to countries where there is no law to protect the social rights and the government tolerates a high level of discrimination against women's social rights. A score of 1 indicates that women have some social rights under law, but that these rights are not effectively enforced and that the government tolerates a moderate level of discrimination against women's social rights. A score of 2 indicates that women have some social rights under law and that the government tolerates a low level of discrimination against women's social rights. A score of 3 indicates that all or nearly all of women's social rights are guaranteed by law and that the government fully and vigorously enforces the law (Cingranelli and Richards 2008).

The scale of the composite measure of women's political, social, and economic rights variable ranges from 0 to 9.

IV. Economic Development

There are mainly two approaches to the concept of economic development. The traditional approach defines development strictly in economic terms. Economic growth is thus measured by the Gross Domestic Product (GDP) or the Gross National Product (GNP) of a country during a specific year.[9] Since the early 1970s, the conventional measure has come under increasing criticism for its inaccurate and misleading measures of economic activities (Nordhaus and Tobin 1971, Weinrobe 1974, Zolotas 1983, Mamalakis 1996, Nordhaus 2000, Smith and Ingham 2005). Smith and Ingham (2005) pointed out that using either GDP or GNP alone to measure economic growth is problematic simply because the traditional measure of economic growth does not necessarily reflect human development or the increased well-being of people and that the measure tends to overstate economic growth and to understate economic income by excluding the value of unpaid work by women. A number of different measures have since been recommended to measure economic development, such as Genuine Progress Indicator (GPI), Gross Sustainable Development Product (GSDP), Gross Environment Sustainable Development Index (GESDI), and Gini index. In recent years, an alternative approach embraced a broader dimension and considered economic development as a process of expanding people's well-being. Beginning in 1990, the United Nations Development Programme (UNDP) introduced Human Development Index (HDI) as an alternative to GDP or GNP.[10] The measure combines income (GDP), educational attainment (literacy), and health (life expectancy).[11]

Bartram, Lewis, Lenton, and Wright (2005) suggested that measures such as access to safe drinking water and sanitation facilities should be used as indicators of economic development. In a study of eight former Soviet Union countries, McKee, Balabanova, Akingbade, Pomerleau, Stickley, Rose, and Haerpfer (2006) used access to safe drinking water and improved sanitation facilities to compare the process of economic development between rural and urban areas. The process

9 Economists tend to use GDP per capita and GNP per capita for the same purpose of providing a rough measure of the relative productivity of a country. Theoretically the results of the calculation of GDP per capita and GNP per capita should be the same except that GNP may be less than GDP if much of the income from a country's production flows to foreign persons or firms.

10 The United Nations 1990 *Human Development Report* defined human development as a "process of enlarging people's choices." (p. 10). The measure ranges from 1.0 (highest level of development) to 0 (lowest level of development). HDI is calculated in three steps. The first step is to identify a measure of deprivation a country suffers in each of the three variables, life expectancy, literacy, and GDP per capita. The second step is to determine average deprivation level; and the third step is to calculate HDI as one minus the average deprivation level.

11 For the proposed model in this research, HDI correlates highly with endogenous variables, such as infant mortality, maternal mortality, and the percentage of children underweight for age.

of urbanization is also considered to be closely associated with levels of economic development. Boserup (1970) argued that a reduction in the proportion of the population engaged in agriculture goes hand in hand with economic development. Moore (1965) pointed out that the first-order consequences of economic development involve a labor force shift from one economic sector to another. As the percentage of the labor force in agriculture decreases, the percentage of people engaged in industry and service sector increases.

The economic development variable, in this study, is accordingly measured by (1) percentage of population urbanized (urban), (2) percentage of population with access to safe water sources (water), and (3) percentage of population using adequate sanitation facilities (sanitation). All economic development indicators are continuous variables.

V. Political Development

Political development refers to the transition from authoritarian governance to a democratic political structure (Ghoshal 2004). Tocqueville (1835) and Marshall (1964) defined political development as a process through which the civil, social, and political rights of the citizens are extended, strengthened, and more fully realized. Gastil (1988) and Vanhanen (1997) conceptualized political development as the levels of political rights and freedoms. Bollen (1980) suggested that political development be defined as the "extent to which the political power of the elites is minimized and that of nonelites is maximized." (p. 372).

A review of the literature in the measurement of political democracy reveals critical concerns. According to Bollen (1990), there are four problems in operationalizing democracy in cross-national studies, namely invalid indicators, subjective indicators, ordinal or dichotomous measures, and the failure to test reliability or validity. At the same time, Bollen cautioned against the use of voter turning out as an indicator of political democracy since turnout can be affected by many things and reflects factors that have little to do with the measurement of political democracy; and a flawed measure may result in "potentially serious policy repercussions." (Bollen 1990: 9). Bollen (1990) further considered political rights and civil liberties to be major dimensions that are closely tied to political democracy.

Based on the conceptual framework and data availability, political development in this study is measured by two variables: (1) political terror scale (terror) and (2) political rights and civil liberty (PRCL). The political terror scale is a graded ordinal scale for measuring human rights violations. Poe, Tate, and Keith (1999) maintained that the political terror scale is the "best currently available" measure of political development in cross-national studies, although the measure may be biased toward those countries that abuse human rights (p. 299). Amnesty International and the US State Department respectively coded the variable in the following way: (1) under a secure rule of law: People are not imprisoned for their views and torture is rare or exceptional. Political murders are extraordinarily rare.

(2) There is a limited amount of imprisonment for nonviolent political activities. However, few are affected and torture and beatings are exceptional. Political murder is rare. (3) There is extensive political imprisonment, or a recent history of such imprisonment. Execution or other political murders and brutality may be common. Unlimited detention, with or without trial for political views, is accepted. (4) The practices of level 3 are expanded to larger numbers. Murders, disappearances, and torture are a common part of life. In spite of its generality, on this level, violence affects primarily those who interest themselves in politics or ideas. And (5) The violence of level 4 (torture, murders) has been extended to the whole population. The leaders of these societies place no limits on the means or the thoroughness with which they pursue personal or ideological goals. The political terror scale (1–10) is a composite of the scales from both Amnesty International and the US State Department. For analysis, the political terror variable is recoded with 10 indicating the secure rule of law and 1 indicating that there is no law to protect the whole population and that there is severe violence present.

The second indicator of political development is political freedom and civil liberty. Political freedom, according to Freedom House (2007), does not include governmental performance per se, but rather the freedoms enjoyed by people. It consists of three dimensions: (1) the freedom to vote freely for distinct alternatives in legitimate elections, (2) the freedom to compete for public office and join political parties and organizations, and (3) the freedom to elect representatives who have a decisive impact on public policies and are accountable to the electorate. The first and the third dimensions consist of three questions, each of which is coded from 0 to 4 with 0 representing the smallest degree and 4, the greatest degree. The second dimension consists of four questions, each of the questions is coded from 0 (smallest degree) to 4 (greatest degree). The political freedom variable ends up with a numerical rating of 40.

The civil liberty variable consists of four dimensions and takes into account the freedoms of expression and belief, associational and organizational rights, rule of law, and personal autonomy without interference from the state. There are three questions for the second dimension of the variable (associational and organizational rights). Each of the rest of the three dimensions consists of four questions that are coded from 0 (smallest degree) to 4 (greatest degree). The variable political freedom and civil liberty is a composite measure of the two variables with a total numerical rating from 0 to 100.

3.3 Data Sources

Data used to test the proposed model are obtained from 137 developing countries (or areas). The classification of developing countries can be found in the *Human Development Report 2007–2008* by the United Nations Development Programme (UNDP 2008) (http://hdr.undp.org/en/media/HDR20072008_en_complete.pdf). The United Nations Fund for Population Activities (UNFPA 2008), the United

Nations Children's Fund (UNICEF 2008), and the United Nations Development Programme (UNDP 2008) provide the majority of the data. Variables and data sources are presented in Table 3.5.

Table 3.5 Variables and Data Sources

Variables	Data Sources
Economic Development (ECOD)	
% population using adequate sanitation facilities	UNFPA. 2008. *The State of the World Population.*
% population using safe water	UNFPA. 2008. *The State of the World Population.*
% population urbanized	UNFPA. 2008. *The State of the World Population.*
Political Development (POLD)	
Political terror scale	Mark Gibney. 2007. Political terror scale.
Political freedom and civil liberty	Freedom House. 2007. *Freedom in the World.*
Maternal-/Child Care (MCHC)	
Skilled attendance at delivery	UNICEF. 2008. *The State of the World's Children.*
Antenatal care coverage	UNICEF. 2008. *The State of the World's Children.*
Children immunized against measles	UNICEF. 2008. *The State of the World's Children.*
Contraceptive prevalence	UNICEF. 2008. *The State of the World's Children.*
Women's Rights (WOMR)	
Abortion rights	Center for Reproductive Rights. 2008. *World Abortion Laws.*
Economic, political and social rights	CIRI. 2008. *CIRI Human Rights Data Project.*
Gender Equality (GEND)	
Female gross secondary enrollment	UNDP. 2008. *Human Development Report 2007–08.*
Estimated female income	UNDP. 2008. *Human Development Report 2007–08.*
Gender equity index	FAFIA-AFAI. 2007. *Social Watch.*
Seats in parliament held by women	UNDP. 2008. *Human Development Report 2007–08.*
Women's Reproductive Health (WORH)	
Infant mortality	UNICEF. 2008. *The State of the World's Children.*
Maternal mortality	UNICEF. 2008. *The State of the World's Children.*
Infant with low birth weight	UNICEF. 2008. *The State of the World's Children.*

Chapter 4
Findings and Analysis

Chapter 4 discusses the empirical findings of the hypothesized model. This chapter is divided into four sections. The first section focuses on the descriptive statistics of the variables. The second section assesses the parameters of the measurement model, in particular the reliability of the variables and the factor loadings on the constructs. The estimates of the structural parameters of the model are presented in the third section. Section four provides discussions on the estimates of the alternative model.

Structural equation modeling (SEM) is used to test the hypothesized model. SEM is a modeling technique that can handle a large number of endogenous and exogenous variables as well as latent (unobserved) variables. It is considered to lend to causal interpretations of observational data (Bollen 1989). The SEM analysis is done in two steps. The first step is to validate the measurement model in which the indicators measure the corresponding latent variables. It is accomplished primarily through confirmatory factor analysis. The second step of the SEM is to test if the pattern of variance and covariance in the data is consistent with the hypothesized structural model. Goodness-of-fit tests and Q-plots are used to determine if the model being tested should be accepted or rejected.

4.1 Descriptive Statistics

Descriptive statistics of the variables is presented in Table 4.1.

Three variables are used to measure economic development (ECOD): percent of population urbanized (urban), percent of population with access to safe water (water), and percent of population using adequate sanitation facilities (sanitation). Approximately 50 percent of the people in developing countries live in urban areas, with Singapore having the highest percentage (100 percent) and Timer-Leste (8 percent) and Bhutan (9 percent) having the lowest percentages. On average, about 78 percent of the population in developing countries has access to safe water. Ethiopia has the lowest percentage (22 percent), followed by Somalia (29 percent). Eleven countries have provided their populations with 100 percent access to safe water. These countries are Barbados, Cyprus, Korea (D), Lebanon, Mauritius, Qatar, Singapore, Tonga, Tuvalu, United Arab Emirates, and Uruguay. On average, about 60 percent of the population in developing countries is provided with adequate sanitation facilities, with Chad and Eritrea having the lowest percentage (9 percent). The following nine countries are found to have provided their people with 100 percent access to adequate sanitation facilities: Bahamas,

Table 4.1 Descriptive Statistics (variable label in parenthesis)

Variables	Mean	Maximum - Minimum	% Missing (N=137)	Skewness
% population using adequate sanitation facilities (sanitation)	60.2734	100 - 9.00	6.569	-.005
% population with access to safe water (water)	77.8605	100 - 22.00	5.839	-.774
% population urbanized (urban)	50.6788	100 - 8.00	0.00	0.274
Political terror scale (terror)	6.4628	10.00 - 2.00	8.759	0.252
Political freedom and civil liberty (prcl)	54.8309	99.00 - 1.00	0.730	-.158
% births attended by skilled health personnel (skilled)	71.3459	100 - 6.00	2.920	-.677
% women aged 15–49 attended at least once during pregnancy by skilled health personnel (antenatal)	80.0593	100 - 16	13.137	-1.393
% one-year old children immunized against measles (measles)	81.5221	99.00 - 23.00	0.730	-1.092
% women aged 15–49 currently using contraception (contraception)	41.8984	87.00 - 3.00	6.569	0.084
Legal abortion right (abortion)	3.5074	8.00 - 1.00	0.730	0.737
Women's economic, political, and social rights (EPS-rights)	4.1278	8.00 - 0	2.920	0.270
Female gross secondary enrollment rate (enroll)	61.6807	113.00* - 7.00	13.138	-.199
Estimated female earned income (income)	3,917.5593	22433.00 - 424.00	13.137	2.255
Gender equity index (gei)	56.6981	84.00 - 31.00	22.627	0.160
% total seats in parliament held by women (seats)	14.5174	45.30 - 0	11.678	0.806
Infant mortality (infant)	52.051	165.00 - 3.00	0.730	0.885
Maternal mortality (maternal)	423.9008	2000 - 1.00	4.379	1.435
% infants with low birth weight (weight)	12.6719	36.00 - 0	6.567	1.205

*Female gross enrolment ratio in excess of 100 indicates that there are pupils or students outside the theoretical age group who are enrolled in that level of education.

Barbados, Cyprus, Qatar, Samoa, Seychelles, Singapore, Trinidad & Tobago, and Uruguay.

Two variables are used to measure political development (POLD): (1) political terror scale (terror) and (2) political freedom and civil liberty (prcl). Afghanistan, Iraq, Nepal, and Sudan are found to have the highest level of political terror, while Chili, Comoros, Grenada, Saint Vincent & Grenadines, Sao Tome & Principe, Uruguay, and Vanuatu score the lowest levels on the scale of political terror. For the variable political freedom and civil liberty, the mean score for the 137 developing countries is 54.83. Barbados has the best record (99) compared with other developing countries. Countries with scores lower than 10 are: North Korea (1), followed by Somalia (4), Cuba (7), Myanmar (7), Libyan Arab Jamahiriya (9), and Syria Arab Republic (9).

In terms of maternal-child care (MCHC), four variables are used: (1) percentage births attended by skilled health personnel (skilled), (2) percentage women aged 15–49 who are attended to by skilled health personnel at least once during pregnancy (antenatal), (3) percentage one-year old children who are immunized against measles (measles), and (4) percentage women aged 15–49 currently using contraception (contraception). On average, about 71 percent of the births in developing countries are attended to by skilled health personnel. The variable ranges from 100 percent to 6 percent with Ethiopia having the lowest percentage (6 percent). Countries with full coverage (100 percent) are Antigua Barbuda, Barbados, Chile, Cuba, Dominica, Grenada, Jordan, Korea (R), Palau, Saint Kitts & Nevis, Saint Vincent & Principe, Samoa, Singapore, Tuvalu, and Uruguay. Concerning antenatal care, about 80 percent of the women aged 15 to 49 in developing countries as a whole have visited skilled health personnel at least once during pregnancy, but only 16 percent of the women in Afghanistan have done so. Countries with 100 percent of women of reproductive age who have received antenatal care are: Antigua Barbuda, Barbados, Brunei Darussalam, Cuba, Dominica, Oman, Saint Kitts & Nevis, and Sri Lanka. On average, almost 82 percent of one-year old children in developing countries have been immunized against measles. The highest percentage of children who have been immunized (99 percent) are found in the following countries: Antigua Barbuda, Argentina, Bahrain, Brazil, Dominican Republic, El Salvador, Grenada, Korea (R), Kuwait, Mongolia, Occupied Palestinian Territory, Panama, Qatar, Saint Kitts & Nevis, Seychelles, Sri Lanka, and Tonga. Only 23 percent of children have been immunized in Chad. In developing countries, on average, about 42 percent of women of reproductive age use contraceptives. Contraceptive prevalence varies considerably from 87 percent in China to only 3 percent in Chad, followed by Sierra Leone (4 percent), Angola (6 percent), Guinea (7 percent), Sudan (7 percent), Eritrea (8 percent), Guinea-Bissau (8 percent), Mauritania (8 percent), and Djibouti (9 percent).

Abortion right (abortion) and women's economic, political, and social rights (EPS-rights) are used to measure women's human rights (WOMR). Countries that have granted women the full legal right to abortion (coded 8) are Bahrain, Cambodia, Cape Verde, China, Cuba, Guyana, Korea (D), Mongolia, Nepal, Singapore, South

Africa, and Vietnam. Countries that have the most restricted abortion policy (coded as 1) are Afghanistan, Antigua Barbuda, Bangladesh, Brunei Darussalam, Côte d'Ivoire, Dominica, Guatemala, Indonésie, Kenya, Kiribati, Lebanon, Libyen Arab Jamahiriya, Malawi, Myanmar, Nigeria, Occupied Palestinian Territory, Papua New Guinea, Paraguay, Solomon Islands, Sri Lanka, Syrian Arab Republic, Tanzania United Republic, Tuvalu, Uganda, United Arab Emirates, Venezuela, and Yemen. The variable, women's economic, political, and social rights range from 0 (no law to protect women's rights) to 8 (nearly all of women's rights are guaranteed by law). Countries with a score of 8 are Argentina, Grenada, and Trinidad & Tobago. Countries that have no law to protect women's human rights are Saudi Arabia (0), followed by Iran (1), Kuwait (1), and Qatar (1).

Four variables are used to measure gender equality: (1) female gross secondary enrollment rate (enroll), (2) estimated female earned income (income), (3) percentage total seats in parliament held by women (seats), and (4) gender equity index (gei). On average, about 62 percent of the women in developing countries have enrolled in secondary schools, but in Niger only 7 percent of women have done so, followed by Chad (8 percent). The highest enrollment rates are found in Bahrain (102 percent), Barbados (103 percent), Brazil (111 percent), Dominica (106 percent), Grenada (102 percent), Guyana (103 percent), Libyan Arab Jamahiriya (107 percent), Occupied Palestinian Territory (102 percent), Seychelles (105 percent), Suriname (100 percent), Tonga (102 percent), and Uruguay (113 percent).[1] The average annual income for women in developing countries as a whole is estimated at $3,917.559. Women in Hong Kong have the highest average annual income ($22,433.00), followed by Singapore ($20,044.00). Yemen and Congo (D) are found to have the lowest average female annual income, only $424.00 and $488.00 respectively. The third indicator of gender equality is the percentage of total seats in parliament held by women. On average, only 14.5 percent of the total seats in parliament are held by women in developing countries. Rwanda has the highest percentage (45.3 percent) and Saudi Arabia (0 percent), Solomon Islands (0 percent), Yemen (0.7 percent), and Papua New Guinea (0.9 percent) have the lowest percentages. For the fourth indicator, gender equity index, Rwanda has the highest score (84), followed by Barbados (80). Yemen is found to have the lowest score (31).

With regard to women's reproductive health indicators, three variables are used: infant mortality, maternal mortality, and percentage infants with low birth weight (infants who weigh less than 2,500 grams). On average, there are 52 infant deaths per 1,000 live births in developing countries. Infant mortality ranges from 3 per 1,000 live births in Singapore to 165 per 1,000 live births in Sierra Leone. There are substantial differences in maternal mortality, from only 1 per 100,000 live births to 2,000 per 100,000 live births. Grenada has the lowest rate; while Sierra Leone, Afghanistan, and Malawi have the highest rates, 2,000, 1,900, and

1 Female gross enrollment rates in excess to 100 indicate that there are students outside the theoretical age groups who are enrolled in that level of education (United Nations Development Programme 2008. *Human Development Report 2007–08*).

1,800 respectively. On average, 13 percent of infants in developing countries as a whole are below normal weight. Thirty-six percent of infants in Bangladesh are below normal weight, followed by Yemen (32 percent), Sudan (31 percent), and India (30 percent).

Table 4.2 Analysis of the Variables

Variables	Statistics	Countries*
% population using adequate sanitation facilities (sanitation)	60–100%	Algeria, Antigua Barbuda, Argentina, Bahamas, Barbados, Bhutan, Brazil, Chile, Columbia, Costa Rica, Cuba, Cyprus, Djibouti, Dominica, Dominican Rep, Ecuador, Egypt, El Salvador, Egypt, El Salvador, Fiji, Grenada, Guatemala, Guyana, Honduras, Iraq, Jamaica, Jordan, Lebanon, Libyan Arab Jamahiriya, Malawi, Malaysia, Marshall Islands, Mauritius, Mexico, Morocco, Myanmar, Occupied Palestinian Territory, Palau, Panama, Paraguay, Peru, Philippines, Qatar, saint Kitts & Nevis, Saint Lucia, Samoa, Seychelles, Singapore, South Africa, Sri Lanka, Suriname, Syrian Arab Rep, Thailand, Tonga, Trinidad & Tobago, Tunisia, Turkey, Tuvalu, United Arab Emirates, Uruguay, Venezuela, Vietnam.
	10–59%	Afghanistan, Angola, Bangladesh, Belize, Benin, Bolivia, Botswana, Burkina Faso, Burundi, Cambodia, Cameroon , Cape Verde, Central African Rep, Chad, China, Comoros, Congo R., Congo D., Cote d'Ivoire, Equatorial Guinea, Ethiopia, Gabon, Gambia, Ghana, Guinea, Guinea-Bissau, Haiti, India, Indonesia, Kenya, Kiribati, Korea (D), Laos, Lesotho, Liberia, Madagascar, Maldives, Mali, Mauritania, Micronesia, Mongolia, Mozambique, Namibia, Nepal, Nicaragua, Niger, Nigeria, Oman, Pakistan, Papua New Guinea, Rwanda, Sao Tome & Principe, Senegal, Sierra Leone, Solomon Islands, Somalia, Sudan, Swaziland, Tanzania United Rep, Timor-Leste, Togo, Uganda, Vanuatu, Yemen, Zambia, Zimbabwe.
	below 10%	Eritrea.
% population using safe water (water)	60–100%	Algeria, Antigua Barbuda, Argentina, Bahamas, Bangladesh, Barbados, Belize, Benin, Bhutan, Bolivia, Botswana, Brazil, Burkina Faso, Burundi, Cameroon , Cape Verde, Central African Rep, Chile, China, Colombia, Comoros, Costa Rica, Cote d'Ivoire, Cuba, Cyprus, Djibouti, Dominica, Dominican Rep, Ecuador, Egypt, El Salvador, Eritrea, Gabon, Gambia, Ghana, Grenada, Guatemala, Guyana, Honduras, India, Indonesia, Iran, Iraq, Jamaica, Jordan, Kenya, Kiribati , Korea (D), Korea (R), Lebanon, Lesotho, Liberia, Malawi, Malaysia, Maldives, Marshall Islands, Mauritius, Mexico, Micronesia, Mongolia, Morocco, Myanmar, Namibia, Nepal, Nicaragua, Occupied Palestinian Territory, Oman, Pakistan, Palau, Panama, Peru, Paraguay, Philippines, Qatar, Rwanda, Saint Kitts & Nevis, Saint Lucia, Samoa, Sao Tome & Principe, Senegal, Seychelles, Sierra Leone, Singapore, Solomon Islands, South Africa, Sri Lanka, Sudan, Swaziland, Syrian Arab Rep, Tanzania United Rep, Thailand, Suriname, Tonga, Trinidad & Tobago, Tuvalu, Uganda, Tunisia, Turkey, United Arab Emirates, Uruguay, Vanuatu, Venezuela, Vietnam, Yemen, Zimbabwe.
	10–59%	Afghanistan, Angola, Cambodia, Chad, Congo R., Congo D., Equatorial Guinea, Ethiopia, Fiji, Guinea, Guinea-Bissau, Haiti, Laos, Madagascar, Mali, Mauritania, Mozambique, Niger, Nigeria, Papua New Guinea, Somalia, Timor-Leste, Togo, Zambia.

Table 4.2 Continued

% population urbanized (urban)	60–100%	Algeria, Argentina, Bahamas, Bahrain, Barbados, Bolivia, Brazil, Brunei Darussalam, Chile, Colombia, Costa Rica, Cuba, Cyprus, Djibouti, Dominica, Dominican Rep, Ecuador, El Salvador, Gabon, Hong Kong, Iran, Iraq, Jordan, Korea (D), Korea (R), Kuwait, Lebanon, Libyan Arab Jamahiriya, Malaysia, Marshall Islands, Mauritania, Mexico, Nauru, Occupied Palestinian Territory, Oman, Peru, Philippines, Qatar, Saint Vincent & Grenadines, Saudi Arabia, Singapore, Suriname, Trinidad & Tobago, Tunisia, Turkey, United Arab Emirates, Uruguay, Venezuela.
	10–59%	Afghanistan, Angola, Antigua Barbuda, Bangladesh, Belize, Benin, Botswana, Burkina Faso, Burundi, Cambodia, Cameroon , Cape Verde, Central African Rep, Chad, China, Comoros, Congo R., Congo D., Cote d'Ivoire, Egypt, Equatorial Guinea, Eritrea, Ethiopia, Fiji, Gambia, Ghana, Grenada, Guatemala, Guinea, Guinea-Bissau, Guyana, Haiti, Honduras, India, Indonesia, Jamaica, Kenya, Kiribati , Laos, Lesotho, Liberia, Madagascar, Malawi, Maldives, Mali, Mauritius, Micronesia, Mongolia, Morocco, Mozambique, Myanmar, Namibia, Nepal, Nicaragua, Niger, Nigeria, Pakistan, Palau, Panama, Papua New Guinea, Paraguay, Rwanda, Saint Kitts & Nevis, Saint Lucia, Samoa, Sao Tome & Principe, Senegal, Seychelles, Sierra Leone, Solomon Islands, Somalia, South Africa, Sri Lanka, Sudan, Swaziland, Syrian Arab Rep, Tanzania United Rep, Thailand, Togo, Tonga, Tuvalu, Uganda, Vanuatu, Vietnam, Yemen, Zambia, Zimbabwe.
	below 10%	Bhutan, Timor-Leste.
Political terror scale (terror)	7–10	Argentina, Bahamas, Bahrain, Barbados, Belize, Benin, Bhutan, Bolivia, Botswana, Brunei Darussalam, Burkina Faso, Cape Verde, Chile, Comoros, Congo (R), Costa Rica, Cote D'Ivoire, Cuba, Cyprus, Djibouti, El Salvador, Fiji, Gabon, Gambia, Ghana, Grenada, Guinea, Guinea-Bissau, Guyana, Jordan, Korea (R), Kuwait, Lesotho, Madagascar, Malaysia, Maldives, Mali, Marshall Islands, Mongolia, Namibia, Niger, Nigeria, Oman, Panama, Paraguay, Peru, Qatar, Rwanda, Saint Lucia, Saint Vincent & Grenadines, Sao Tome & Principe, Senegal, Seychelles, Sierra Leone, Singapore, Solomon Islands, Suriname, Swaziland, Tunisia, United Arab Emirates, Uruguay, Vanuatu.
	0–6	Afghanistan, Algeria, Angola, Bangladesh, Brazil, Burundi, Cambodia, Cameroon, central African Rep, Chad, China, Columbia, Congo (D), Dominica, Ecuador, Egypt, Equatorial Guinea, Eritrea, Ethiopia, Guatemala, Haiti, Honduras, India, Indonesia, Iran, Iraq, Jamaica, Kenya, Laos, Lebanon, Liberia, Libyan Arab Jamahiriya, Malawi, Mexico, Morocco, Mozambique, Myanmar, Nepal, Nigeria, Occupied Palestinian Territory, Pakistan, Papua New Guinea, Philippines, Saudi Arabia, Somalia, South Africa, Sri Lanka, Sudan, Syrian United Rep, Tanzania United Rep, Thailand, Togo, Trinidad & Tobago, Turkey, Uganda, Venezuela, Yemen, Zambia, Zimbabwe.

Table 4.2 Continued

Political freedom and civil liberty (PRCL)	60–100	Antigua Barbuda, Argentina, Bahamas, Barbados, Belize, Benin, Bolivia, Botswana, Brazil, Cape Verde, Chile, Colombia, Comoros, Costa Rica, Cyprus, Dominica, Dominican Rep, Ecuador, El Salvador, Ghana, Grenada, Guyana, Honduras, Hong Kong, India, Indonesia, Jamaica, Kenya, Kiribati, Korea (R), Lesotho, Mali, Marshall Islands, Mauritius, Mexico, Micronesia, Mongolia, Namibia, Nauru, Palau, Panama, Papua New Guinea, Paraguay, Peru, Philippines, Saint Kitts & Nevis, Saint Lucia, Saint Vincent & Grenadines, Samoa, Sao Tome & Principe, Senegal, Seychelles, Sierra Leone, Solomon Islands, South Africa, Suriname, Trinidad & Tobago, Turkey, Tuvalu, Uruguay, Vanuatu.
	10–59	Afghanistan, Algeria, Angola, Bahrain, Bangladesh, Bhutan, Brunei Darussalam, Burkina Faso, Burundi, Cambodia, Cameroon, Central African Rep, Chad, China, Congo (R), Congo (D), Cote D'Ivoire, Djibouti, Egypt, equatorial Guinea, Eritrea, Ethiopia, Fiji, Gabon, Gambia, Guatemala, Guinea, Guinea-Bissau, Haiti, Iran, Iraq, Jordan, Kuwait, Laos, Lebanon, Liberia, Madagascar, Malawi, Malaysia, Maldives, Mauritania, Morocco, Mozambique, Nepal, Nigeria, Occupied Palestinian Territory, Oman, Pakistan, Qatar, Rwanda, Saudi Arabia, Singapore, Sri Lanka, Sudan, Swaziland, Tanzania United Rep, Thailand, Timor-Leste, Togo, Tonga, Tunisia, Uganda, United Arab Emirates, Venezuela, Vietnam, Yemen, Zambia, Zimbabwe.
	below 10	Cuba, Korea (D), Libyan Arab Jamahiriya, Myanmar, Somalia, Syrian Arab Rep.
Skilled attendance at delivery (skilled)	60–100%	Algeria, Antigua Barbuda, Argentina, Bahamas, Bahrain, Barbados, Belize, Benin, Bolivia, Botswana, Brazil, Brunei Darussalam, Cameroon, Cape Verde, Chile, China, Colombia, Comoros, Congo (R), Congo (D), Costa Rica, Cote D'Ivoire, Cuba, Djibouti, Dominica, Dominican Rep, Ecuador, Egypt, El Salvador, Equatorial Guinea, Fiji, Gabon, Grenada, Guyana, Indonesia, Iran, Iraq, Jamaica, Jordan, Kiribati, Korea (D), Korea (R), Kuwait, Lebanon, Libyan Arab Jamahiriya, Malaysia, Maldives, Marshall Islands, Mauritius, Mexico, Micronesia, Mongolia, Morocco, Namibia, Nicaragua, Occupied Palestinian Territory, Oman, Palau, Panama, Paraguay, Peru, Philippines, Qatar, Saint Kitts & Nevis, Saint Lucia, Saint Vincent & Grenadines, Samoa, Sao Tome & Principe, Saudi Arabia, Singapore, Solomon Islands, South Africa, Sri Lanka, Sudan, Suriname, Swaziland, Syrian Arab Rep, Thailand, Togo, Tonga, Trinidad & Tobago, Tunisia Turkey, Tuvalu, United Arab Emirates, Uruguay, Vanuatu, Venezuela, Vietnam, Zimbabwe.
	10–59%	Afghanistan, Angola, Bangladesh, Bhutan, Burkina Faso, Burundi, Cambodia, Central African Rep, Chad, Eritrea, Gambia, Ghana, Guatemala, Guinea, Guinea-Bissau, Haiti, Honduras, India, Kenya, Laos, Lesotho, Liberia, Madagascar, Malawi, Mali, Mauritania, Mozambique, Myanmar, Nepal, Niger, Nigeria, Pakistan, Papua New Guinea, Rwanda, Senegal, Sierra Leone, Somalia, Tanzania United Rep, Timor-Leste, Uganda, Yemen, Zambia.
	below 10%	Ethiopia.

Table 4.2 Continued

Antenatal care coverage (antenatal)	60–100%	Algeria, Angola, Antigua Barbuda, Argentina, Bahrain, Barbados, Belize, Benin, Bolivia, Botswana, Brazil, Brunei Darussalam, Burkina, Burundi, Cameroon, Cape Verde, Central African Rep, Chile, China, Colombia, Comoros, Congo (R), Congo (D), Costa Rica, Cote D'Ivoire, Cuba, Djibouti, Dominica, Dominican Rep, Ecuador, Egypt, El Salvador, Equatorial Guinea, Eritrea, Gabon, Gambia, Ghana, Grenada, Guatemala, Guinea, Guinea-Bissau, Guyana, Haiti, Honduras, India, Indonesia, Iran, Iraq, Jamaica, Jordan, Kenya, Kiribati, Kuwait, Lebanon, Lesotho, Liberia, Libyan Arab Jamahiriya, Madagascar, Malawi, Malaysia, Maldives, Mauritania, Mexico, Mongolia, Morocco, Mozambique, Myanmar, Namibia, Nicaragua, Occupied Palestinian Territory, Oman, Panama, Papua New Guinea, Paraguay, Peru, Philippines, Rwanda, Saint Kitts & Nevis, Saint Vincent & Grenadines, Sao Tome & Principe, Saudi Arabia, Senegal, Sierra Leone, South Africa, Sri Lanka, Sudan, Suriname, Swaziland, Syrian Arab Rep, Tanzania United Rep, Thailand, Timor-Leste, Togo, Trinidad & Tobago, Tunisia Turkey, Uganda, United Arab Emirates, Uruguay, Venezuela, Vietnam, Zambia, Zimbabwe.
	10–59%	Afghanistan, Bangladesh, Bhutan, Cambodia, Chad, Ethiopia, Laos, Mali, Nepal, Niger, Nigeria, Pakistan, Saint Lucia, Somalia, Yemen.
Children immunized against measles (measles)	60–100%	Afghanistan, Algeria, Antigua Barbuda, Argentina, Bahamas, Bahrain, Bangladesh, Barbados, Belize, Benin, Bhutan, Bolivia, Botswana, Brazil, Brunei Darussalam, Burkina Faso, Burundi, Cambodia, Cameroon, Cape Verde, Chile, China, Colombia, Comoros, Congo (D), Costa Rica, Cuba, Cyprus, Djibouti, Dominica, Dominican Rep, Ecuador, Egypt, El Salvador, Eritrea, Fiji, Gambia, Ghana, Grenada, Guatemala, Guinea-Bissau, Guyana, Honduras, Indonesia, Iran, Iraq, Jamaica, Jordan, Kenya, Korea (D), Korea (R), Kuwait, Lebanon, Lesotho, Liberia, Libyan Arab Jamahiriya, Malawi, Malaysia, Maldives, Mali, Marshall Islands, Mauritania, Mauritius, Mexico, Micronesia, Mongolia, Morocco, Mozambique, Myanmar, Namibia, Nauru, Nepal, Nicaragua, Niger, Occupied Palestinian Territory, Oman, Pakistan, Palau, Panama, Papua New Guinea, Paraguay, Peru, Philippines, Qatar, Rwanda, Saint Kitts & Nevis, Saint Lucia, Saint Vincent & Grenadines, Sao Tome & Principe, Saudi Arabia, Senegal, Seychelles, Sierra Leone, Singapore, Solomon Islands, South Africa, Sri Lanka, Sudan, Suriname, Swaziland, Syrian Arab rep, Tanzania United rep, Thailand, Togo, Tonga, Trinidad & Tobago, Tunisia, Turkey, Tuvalu, Uganda, United Arab Emirates, Uruguay, Vanuatu, Venezuela, Vietnam, Yemen, Zambia, Zimbabwe.
	10–59%	Angola, Central African rep, Chad, Congo (R), Cote D'Ivoire, Equatorial Guinea, Ethiopia, Gabon, Guinea, Haiti, India, Kiribati, Laos, Madagascar, Nigeria, Samoa, Somalia, Timor-Leste.
Contraceptive prevalence (contraception)	60–100%	Bahrain, China, Colombia, Costa Rica, Cuba, Dominican Rep, Ecuador, El Salvador, Honduras, Iran, Jamaica, Korea (D), Korea (R), Mauritius, Mexico, Mongolia, Morocco, Nicaragua, Paraguay, Peru, Singapore, South Africa, Sri Lanka, Tunisia, Turkey, Uruguay, Venezuela, Vietnam.

Table 4.2 Continued

	10–59%	Afghanistan, Algeria, Antigua Barbuda, Argentina, Bangladesh, Barbados, Belize, Benin, Bhutan, Bolivia, Botswana, Brazil, Burkina Faso, Burundi, Cambodia, Cameroon, Cape Verde, Central African Rep, Chile, Comoros, Congo (R), Congo (D), Cote D'Ivoire, Dominica, Dominican Rep, Egypt, Ethiopia, Fiji, Gabon, Gambia, Ghana, Grenada, Guatemala, Guyana, Haiti, India, Indonesia, Iraq, Jordan, Kenya, Kiribati, Laos, Lebanon, Lesotho, Liberia, Libyan Arab Jamahiriya, Madagascar, Malawi, Malaysia, Maldives, Marshall Islands, Micronesia, Mozambique, Myanmar, Namibia, Nepal, Niger, Nigeria, Occupied Palestinian Territory, Oman, Pakistan, Palau, Papua New Guinea, Philippines, Qatar, Rwanda, Saints Kitts & Nevis, Saint Lucia, Saint Vincent & Grenadines, Samoa, Sao Tome & Principe, Saudi Arabia, Senegal, Solomon Islands, Suriname, Swaziland, Syrian Arab Rep, Tanzania United Rep, Thailand, Timor-Leste, Togo, Tonga, Trinidad& Tobago, Tuvalu, Uganda, United Arab Emirates, Vanuatu, Yemen, Zambia, Zimbabwe.
	below 10%	Angola, Djibouti, Guinea, Guinea-Bissau, Mali, Mauritania, Sierra Leone, Sudan.
Legal abortion right (abortion)	5–8	Bahrain, Barbados, Belize, Benin, Botswana, Burkina Faso, Cambodia, Cape Verde, China, Colombia, Cuba, Cyprus, Ethiopia, Fiji, Ghana, Guinea, Guyana, Hong Kong, India, Korea (D), Korea(R), Liberia, Mongolia, Namibia, Nepal, Saint Lucia, Saint Vincent & Grenadines, Seychelles, Singapore, South Africa, Swaziland, Thailand, Togo, Tunisia, Turkey, Vietnam.
	0–4	Afghanistan, Algeria, Angola, Antigua Barbuda, Argentina, Bahamas, Bangladesh, Bhutan, Bolivia, Brazil, Brunei Darussalam, Burundi, Cameroon, Central African Rep, Chad, Chile, Comoros, Congo (R), Congo (D), Costa Rica, Cote D'Ivoire, Djibouti, Dominica, Dominican Rep, Ecuador, Egypt, El Salvador, Equatorial Guinea, Eritrea, Gabon, Gambia, Grenada, Guatemala, Guinea Bissau, Haiti, Honduras, Indonesia, Iran, Iraq, Jamaica, Jordan, Kenya, Kiribati, Kuwait, Laos, Lebanon, Lesotho, Libyan Arab Jamahiriya, Madagascar, Malawi, Malaysia, Maldives, Mali, Marshall Islands, Mauritania, Mauritius, Mexico, Micronesia, Morocco, Mozambique, Myanmar, Nauru, Nicaragua, Niger, Nigeria, Occupied Palestinian Territory, Oman, Pakistan, Palau, Panama, Papua New Guinea, Paraguay, Peru, Philippines, Qatar, Rwanda, Saint Kitts & Nevis, Samoa, Sao Tome & Principe, Saudi Arabia, Senegal, Sierra Leone, Solomon Islands, Somalia, Sri Lanka, Sudan, Suriname, Syrian Arab Rep, Tanzania United Rep, Tonga, Trinidad & Tobago, Tuvalu, Uganda, United Arab Emirates, Uruguay, Vanuatu, Venezuela, Yemen, Zambia, Zimbabwe.
Women's economic, political, and social rights (EPS-rights)	5–9	Antigua Barbuda, Argentina, Barbados, Belize, Bhutan, Brazil, Cambodia, Chile, Costa Rica, Cuba, Cyprus, El Salvador, Eritrea, Fiji, Grenada, Guatemala, Guyana, Honduras, Iraq, Jamaica, Korea (R), Laos, Madagascar, Marshall Islands, Mauritania, Mauritius, Mexico, Mongolia, Morocco, Mozambique, Namibia, Oman, Palau, Panama, Paraguay, Peru, Rwanda, Saints Kitts & Nevis, Saint Vincent & Grenadines, Samoa, Seychelles, Singapore, South Africa, Thailand, Trinidad & Tobago, Uruguay, Venezuela, Vietnam.

Table 4.2 Continued

	0–4	Afghanistan, Algeria, Angola, Bahamas, Bahrain, Bangladesh, Benin, Bolivia, Botswana, Brunei Darussalam, Burkina Faso, Burundi, Cameroon, Cape Verde, Central African Rep, Chad, China, Colombia, Comoros, Congo (R), Congo (D), Cote D'Ivoire, Djibouti, Dominica, Dominican rep, Ecuador, Egypt, Equatorial Guinea, Ethiopia, Gabon, Gambia, Ghana, Guinea, Guinea-Bissau, India, Indonesia, Iran, Jordan, Kenya, Kiribati, Korea (D), Kuwait, Lebanon, Lesotho, Liberia, Libyan Arab Jamahiriya, Malawi, Malaysia, Maldives, Mali, Myanmar, Nauru, Nepal, Nicaragua, Niger, Nigeria, Pakistan, Papua New Guinea, Philippines, Qatar, Saint Lucia, Sao Tome & Principe, Saudi Arabia, Senegal, Sierra Leone, Solomon Islands, Somalia, Sri Lanka, Sudan, Suriname, Swaziland, Syrian United Rep, Tanzania United Rep, Togo, Tonga, Tunisia, Turkey, Tuvalu, Uganda, United Arab Emirates, Vanuatu, Yemen, Zambia, Zimbabwe.
Female gross secondary enrollment (enroll)	60–113%	Algeria, Argentina, Bahamas, Bahrain, Belize, Bolivia, Botswana, Brazil, Brunei Darussalam, Cape Verde, Chile, China, Colombia, Costa Rica, Cuba, Cyprus, Dominica, Dominican Rep, Ecuador, Egypt, El Salvador, Fiji, Grenada, Guyana, Honduras, Hong Kong, Indonesia, Iran, Jamaica, Jordan, Korea (R), Kuwait, Lebanon, Libyan Arab Jamahiriya, Malaysia, Maldives, Mauritius, Mexico, Mongolia, Namibia, Nicaragua, Occupied Palestinian Territory, Oman, Panama, Paraguay, Peru, Philippines, Qatar, Saint Kitts & Nevis, Saint Lucia, Saint Vincent & Grenadines, Samoa, Saudi Arabia, Seychelles, South Africa, Sri Lanka, Suriname, Syrian Arab Rep, Thailand, Tonga, Trinidad & Tobago, Tunisia, Turkey, United Arab Emirates, Uruguay, Venezuela, Vietnam.
	10–59%	Angola, Bangladesh, Barbados, Benin, Burkina Faso, Burundi, Cambodia, Cameroon, Comoros, Congo (R), Congo (D), Cote D'Ivoire, Djibouti, Equatorial Guinea, Eritrea, Ethiopia, Gabon, Gambia, Ghana, Guatemala, Guinea, Guinea-Bissau, India, Kenya, Mali, Mauritania, Morocco, Mozambique, Myanmar, Nepal, Nigeria, Pakistan, Papua New Guinea, Rwanda, Sao Tome & Principe, Senegal, Sierra Leone, Solomon Islands, Sudan, Swaziland, Timor-Leste, Togo, Uganda, Vanuatu, Yemen, Zambia, Zimbabwe.
	below 10%	Chad, Niger.
Estimated female income (income)	$4,000 or more	Argentina, Bahamas, Bahrain, Barbados, Belize, Botswana, Brazil, Brunei Darussalam , Chile, China, Colombia, Costa Rica, Cuba, Cyprus, Dominican Rep, Equatorial Guinea, Gabon, Hong Kong, Iran, Korea (R), Kuwait, Libyan Arab Jamahiriya, Malaysia, Mauritius, Mexico, Namibia, Oman, Palau, Panama, Qatar, Saint Lucia, Saint Vincent & Grenadines, Saudi Arabia, Singapore, South Africa, Suriname, Thailand, Tonga, Trinidad & Tobago, Turkey, United Arab Emirates, Uruguay, Venezuela.
	$1,000–3,999	Argentina, Angola, Bangladesh, Bhutan, Bolivia, Cambodia, Cameroon, Cape Verde, Chad, Comoros, Djibouti, Ecuador, Egypt, El Salvador, Fiji, Gambia, Ghana, Guatemala, Guinea, Guyana, Haiti, Honduras, India, Indonesia, Jamaica, Jordan, Kenya, Laos, Lebanon, Lesotho, Maldives, Mauritania, Mongolia, Morocco, Mozambique, Nepal, Nicaragua, Pakistan, Papua New Guinea, Paraguay, Philippines, Rwanda, Samoa, Sao Tome & Principe, Swaziland, Solomon Islands, Sri Lanka, Swaziland, Syrian Arab Rep, Tunisia, Uganda, Vanuatu, Vietnam, Zimbabwe.

Table 4.2 Continued

	below $1,000	Benin, Burkina Faso, Burundi, Central African Rep, Congo (R), Congo (D), Cote D'Ivoire, Eritrea, Ethiopia, Guinea-Bissau, Madagascar, Malawi, Mali, Niger, Nigeria, Sierra Leone, Sudan, Tanzania United Rep, Togo, Yemen, Zambia.
Gender equity index (GEI)	60–100	Argentina, Bahamas, Barbados, Belize, Bolivia, Botswana, Brazil, Burundi, Cambodia, Cape Verde, Chile, China, Columbia, Costa Rica, Cuba, Cyprus, Dominican Rep, Ecuador, Guyana, Honduras, Hong Kong, Jamaica, Kenya, Lesotho, Madagascar, Malawi, Maldives, Mexico, Mongolia, Mozambique, Namibia, Panama, Paraguay, Peru, Philippines, Rwanda, Saint Vincent & Grenadines, South Africa, Suriname, Tanzania United Rep, Thailand, Trinidad & Tobago, Uganda, Uruguay, Venezuela, Vietnam.
	31–59	Algeria, Angola, Bahrain, Bangladesh, Benin, Burkina Faso, Cameroon, Central African Rep, Chad, Congo(R), Congo(D), Cote D'Ivoire, Djibouti, Egypt, Eritrea, Ethiopia, Fiji, Gabon, Gambia, Ghana, Guatemala, Guinea, Guinea-Bissau, Indonesia, Iran, Jordan, Korea (R), Kuwait, Laos, Lebanon, Mali, Mauritius, Morocco, Nepal, Nicaragua, Niger, Nigeria, Oman, Pakistan, Qatar, Saint Lucia, Samoa, Sao Tome & Principe, Saudi Arabia, Senegal, Serra Leone, Solomon Islands, Sri Lanka, Swaziland, Syrian Arab Rep, Togo, Tunisia, Turkey, United Arab Emirates, Vanuatu, Yemen, Zambia, Zimbabwe.
Seats in parliament held by women (seats)	30% or higher	Argentina, Burundi, Costa Rica, Cuba, Guyana, Mozambique, Rwanda, South Africa, Tanzania United Rep.
	15–29%	Angola, Bahamas, Bangladesh, Barbados, Bolivia, Cape Verde, China, Dominican Rep, Ecuador, El Salvador, Equatorial Guinea, Eritrea, Ethiopia, Grenada, Guinea, Honduras, Laos, Lesotho, Mauritius, Mexico, Micronesia, Namibia, Nicaragua, Pakistan, Panama, Peru, Philippines, Saint Lucia, Saint Vincent & Grenadines, Senegal, Seychelles, Sierra Leone, Singapore, Suriname, Swaziland, Timor-Leste, Trinidad & Tobago, Uganda, Venezuela, Vietnam, Zambia, Zimbabwe.
	below 15%	Algeria, Antigua Barbuda, Bahrain, Belize, Benin, Bhutan, Botswana, Brazil, Burkina Faso, Cambodia, Cameroon, Central African Rep, Chad, Chile, Columbia, Comoros, Congo (R), Congo (D), Cote D'Ivoire, Cyprus, Djibouti, Dominica, Egypt, Fiji, Gabon, Gambia, Ghana, Guatemala, Guinea-Bissau, Haiti, India, Indonesia, Iran, Jamaica, Jordan, Kenya, Korea (R), Kuwait, Lebanon, Libyan Arab Jamahiriya, Madagascar, Malawi, Malaysia, Maldives, Mali, Mongolia, Nepal, Nicaragua, Niger, Oman, Papua New Guinea, Paraguay, Qatar, Saint Kitts & Nevis, Samoa, Sao Tome & Principe, Saudi Arabia, Solomon Islands, Sri Lanka, Sudan, Syrian Arab Rep, Thailand, Togo, Tonga, Turkey, United Arab Emirates, Uruguay, Vanuatu, Yemen.
Infant mortality per 1,000 live births (infant)	70–165	Afghanistan, Angola, Benin, Botswana, Burkina Faso, Burundi, Cambodia, Cameroon, Central Africa, Chad, Congo (R), Congo (D), Cote d'Ivoire, Djibouti, Equatorial Guinea, Ethiopia, Gambia, Guinea, Guinea-Bissau, Haiti, Iraq, Kenya, Lesotho, Liberia, Madagascar, Malawi, Mali, Mauritania, Mozambique, Myanmar, Niger, Nigeria, Pakistan, Rwanda, Sao Tome,& Principe, Senegal, Sierra Leone, Somalia, Swaziland, Togo, Uganda, Yemen, Zambia, Zimbabwe.

Table 4.2 Continued

	11–69	Algeria, Antigua Barbuda, Argentina, Bahamas, Bangladesh, Barbados, Belize, Bhutan, Bolivia, Brazil, Cape Verde, China, Colombia, Comoros, Costa Rica, Dominica, Dominican Rep, Ecuador, Egypt, El Salvador, Eritrea, Fiji, Gabon, Ghana, Grenada, Guatemala, Guyana, Honduras, India, Indonesia, Iran, Jamaica, Jordan, Kiribati, Korea (D), Laos, Lebanon, Libyan Arab Jamahiriya, Malaysia, Maldives, Marshall Islands, Mauritius, Mexico, Mongolia, Morocco, Namibia, Nauru, Nepal, Nicaragua, Occupied Palestinian Territory, Oman, Palau, Panama, Papua New Guinea, Paraguay, Peru, Philippines, Qatar, Saint Kitts & Nevis, Saint Lucia, Saint Vincent & Grenadines, Samoa, Saudi Arabia, Seychelles, Solomon Islands, South Africa, Sri Lanka, Sudan, Suriname, Syrian Arab Rep, Thailand, Timor-Leste, Tonga, Trinidad & Tobago, Tunisia, Turkey, Tuvalu, Uruguay, Vanuatu, Venezuela, Vietnam.
	below 10	Bahrain, Brunei Darussalam, Chile, Cuba, Cyprus, Korea (R), Kuwait, Singapore, United Arab Emirates,
Maternal mortality per 100,000 live births (maternal)	1,000–2,000	Afghanistan, Angola, Burkina Faso, Burundi, Central African Rep. Chad, Eritrea, Guinea-Bissau, Kenya, Malawi, Mali, Mauritania, Mozambique, Niger, Rwanda, Sierra Leone, Somalia, Tanzania United Rep, Zimbabwe.
	100–999	Algeria, Bangladesh, Belize, Benin, Bhutan, Bolivia, Botswana, Brazil, Cambodia, Cameroon, Cape Verde, Columbia, Comoros, Congo (R), Congo (D), Cote d'Ivoire, Dominican Rep, Ecuador, El Salvador, Equatorial Guinea, Gabon, Gambia, Ghana, Guatemala, Guinea, Guyana, Haiti, Honduras, India, Indonesia, Iraq, Laos, Lebanon, Lesotho, Liberia, Madagascar, Maldives, Micronesia, Mongolia, Morocco, Myanmar, Namibia, Nepal, Nicaragua, Nigeria, Occupied Palestinian Territory, Pakistan, panama, Papua New Guinea, Paraguay, Peru, Philippines, Qatar, Saint Kitts & Nevis, Samoa, Sao Tome & Principe, Senegal, Solomon Islands, South Africa, Sudan, Suriname, Swaziland, Syrian Arab Rep, Timor-Leste, Togo, Trinidad & Tobago, Tunisia, Uganda, Vietnam, Yemen, Zambia.
	below 100	Antigua Barbuda, Argentina, Bahamas, Bahrain, Barbados, Brunei Darussalam, Chile, China, Costa Rica, Cuba, Cyprus, Dominica, Egypt, Fiji, Grenada, Iran, Jamaica, Jordan, Kiribati, Korea (D), Korea ®, Kuwait, Libyan Arab Jamahiriya, Malaysia, Mauritius, Mexico, Oman, Saint Lucia, Saint Vincent & Grenadines, Saudi Arabia, Seychelles, Singapore, Sri Lanka, Thailand, Turkey, United Arab Emirates, Uruguay, Venezuela.
Infant with low birth weight (weight)	11–36%	Angola, Bangladesh, Barbados, Benin, Bhutan, Botswana, Brunei Darussalam, Burkina, Faso, Burundi, Cambodia, Cameroon, Cape Verde, Central African Rep. Chad, Comoros, Congo (D), Cote D'Ivoire, Djibouti, Dominica, Dominican Rep, Ecuador, Egypt, Equatorial Guinea, Eritrea, Ethiopia, Fiji, Gabon, Gambia, Ghana, Guatemala, Guinea, Guinea-Bissau, Guyana, Haiti, Honduras, India, Iraq, Jamaica, Jordan, Kenya, Laos, Lesotho, Madagascar, Malawi, Maldives, Mali, Marshall Islands, Mauritius, Micronesia, Morocco, Mozambique, Myanmar, Namibia, Nepal, Nicaragua, Niger, Nigeria, Pakistan, Panama, Papua New Guinea, Peru, Philippines, Qatar, saint Lucia, Saint Vincent & Grenadines, Sao Tome & Principe, Saudi Arabia, Senegal, Sierra Leone, Solomon Islands, South Africa, Sri Lanka, Sudan, Suriname, Tanzania United Rep, Timor-Leste, Togo, Trinidad & Tobago, Turkey, Uganda, United Arab Emirates, Yemen, Zambia, Zimbabwe.

Table 4.2 Concluded

	below 10%	Algeria, Antigua Barbuda, Argentina, Bahamas, Bahrain, Belize, Bolivia, Brazil, Chile, China, Columbia, Costa Rica, Cuba, El Salvador, Grenada, Indonesia, Iran, Kiribati, Korea (R), Korea (D), Kuwait, Lebanon, Libyan Arab Jamahiriya, Malaysia, Mexico, Mongolia, Occupied Palestinian Territory, Oman, Palau, Paraguay, Rwanda, Saints Kitts & Nevis, Samoa, Singapore, Swaziland, Syrian Arab Rep, Thailand, Tonga, Tunisia, Tuvalu, Uruguay, Vanuatu, Venezuela, Vietnam.

* Due to missing data, the total number of countries may not add up to 137.

Table 4.2 provides the summary analysis of all of the variables used in this study.

4.2 Measurement Model

This section focuses on the evaluation of the adequacy of the measurement model. To estimate the parameters of the measurement model, confirmatory factor analysis (CFA) is used. CFA seeks to determine if the indicator variables load as predicted on the expected number of factors. That is to say, each proposed indicator is analyzed for its relative contribution toward explaining the variance associated with the changes in the latent factors (economic development, political development, maternal-child care, women's human rights, gender equality, and women's reproductive health). A high level of correlation among the variables that are theoretically related to the constructs indicates convergent validity (Carmine and Zeller 1979, Cook and Campbell 1979). Table 4.3 presents the findings of the measurement model.

Each latent factor shares a scale of 1 with one of its indicators. All factor loadings are statistically significant and highly correlated with the hypothesized latent dimensions. Squared multiple correlations (SMC) are also used to estimate the reliability of the observed variables with their constructs. For example, SMC for the variable percentage urban (urban) is 0.4709, which means that about 47 per cent of the variance in economic development can be explained by percentage urban. Terror scale (terror) and political rights-civil liberty (prcl) respectively account for 60 percent and 23 percent of the total variance in political development. In the same manner, about 71 percent of the variance in maternal-child care can be explained by the variable, percentage births attended to by skilled health personnel (skilled) (SMC=0.7099). Antenatal care (antenatal) and contraceptive use (contraception) account for 36 percent and 57 percent of the variance in maternal-child care respectively. Abortion right (abortion) and women's economic-political-social rights (eps-rights) respectively account for 23 percent and 26 percent of the variance in women's human rights. Estimated female earned income (income) accounts for about 65 percent of the total variance in gender

Table 4.3 Measurement Model Parameters (standardized solution in parentheses)

Variables **Latent Observed**	**Slope**	**SMC**	**Variables** **Latent Observed**	**Slope**	**SMC**
Economic development (ECOD)			Maternal-Child care (MCHC)		
Sanitation	1.0000	0.7159	Skilled	1.0000	0.7099
	(0.8461)			(0.8426)	
Water	0.9711**	0.6906	Antenatal	0.7136**	0.3621
	(0.8311)			(0.6018)	
Urban	0.8183**	0.4709	Measles	0.7925**	0.4368
	(0.6862)			(0.6609)	
			Contraception	0.8969**	0.5724
				(0.7566)	
Political development (POLD)			Women's right (WOMR)		
Terror	1.0000	0.6041	Abortion	1.0000	0.2316
	(0.7772)			(0.4812)	
PRCL	0.6040**	0.2265	EPS-Rights	0.9590**	0.2645
	(0.4759)			(0.5143)	
			Gender equality (GEND)		
			Enroll	1.0000	0.9115
				(0.9548)	
			Income	0.7747**	0.6457
				(0.7973)	
			GEI	0.3845**	0.1693
				(0.4115)	
			Seats	0.0586	0.0038
				(0.0616)	
			Women's reproductive health (WORH)		
			Infant	1.0000	0.6868
				(0.8287)	
			Maternal	0.9601**	0.6331
				(0.7957)	
			Weight	0.6516**	0.2860
				(0.5348)	
GFI=0.921					
AGFI=0.840					
RMSR=0.049					

**: $p<0.01$

equality (SMC=0.6457); and about 91 percent of the variance in gender equality can be explained by the variable, female gross secondary enrollment rate (enroll). About 69 percent of the variance in women's reproductive health can be explained by infant mortality (infant) (SMC=0.6868). Maternal mortality (maternal) and the percentage infants with low birth weight (weight) respectively account for 63 percent and 29 percent of total variance in women's reproductive health. Only one indicator, percentage seats in parliament held by women, has reliability coefficient less than 0.4. This indicator is retained for substantive grounds. To determine whether the presence of the poor indicator results in changes in the values of the measurement model parameters, the measurement model was re-estimated after the one indicator (percentage seats in parliament held by women) was dropped. The value of the factor loading and the R-squared value in the two measurement models are similar.

In sum, results from the confirmatory factor analysis have provided reasonable empirical evidence of the construct validity of the proposed latent traits that are hypothesized to be associated with the selected indicators. In the next section, I'll discuss the test of the hypotheses.

4.3 Structural Model

The third step is to test the hypotheses. The structural portion of the model consists of the relations among latent variables. Table 4.4 presents the coefficients from the estimation of the hypothesized structural equation model.

Table 4.4 Structural Model, LISREL Estimates (Standardized estimates in parentheses)

Endogenous Factors	**Exogenous Factors**				
	ECOD	POLD	MCHC	WOMR	GEND
MCHC	0.9104**	0.0589	-----	-----	-----
	(0.9700)	(0.0479)			
WOMR	0.0700	0.7962**	-----	-----	-----
	(0.0911)	(0.8782)			
GEND	0.9455**	0.0928	-----	-----	-----
	(0.8864)	(0.0667)			
WORH	-----	-----	-.4848**	-.0229	-.4755**
			(-.4799)+	(-.0166)+	(-.5308)+
GFI=0.790					
AGFI=0.700					
RMSR=0.075					

**: $p<0.01$

+: The negative sign "-" indicates that an increase in MCHC, WOMR, and GEND leads to an improvement in women's reproductive health. The discussion on the coding of women's reproductive health indicators can be found in Chapter 3.

Empirical findings indicate the importance of gender equality (GEND) and maternal-child care (MCHC) in explaining women's reproductive health (WORH). The effect of gender equality and maternal-child care on women's reproductive health is strong and statistically significant ($p<0.01$). Economic development (ECOD) is found to be significantly related to gender equality and maternal-child care ($p<.01$). The hypothesized relationship between political development (POLD) and women's human rights (WOMR) is supported. The relationship between women's human rights and reproductive health is not statistically significant.

First, the empirical findings from the 137 developing countries in this study demonstrate that gender equality has a pivotal role to play in the promotion of women's reproductive health. It is noteworthy that the accomplishment of women's reproductive health depends on an undertaking to increase women's social, economic, and political clout, to challenge the prevailing social norms, and to create an environment to advance the gender equality agenda. This finding undercores the importance to enhance the link between gender equality and reproductive health as a global strategy to improve women's reproductive health.

Second, the relationship between women's reproductive health and maternal-child care is found to be strong and statistically significant. This finding, however, is not quite consistent with the ICPD's statement that the attainment of women's reproductive health is not a function of reproductive health programs or access to services per se. The finding from the 137 developing countries in this study may permit a probable verification of the relationship between women's reproductive health and maternal-child care measures.

According to the World Health Organization (WHO 2005, 2009), about 530,000 women die each year in pregnancy or childbirth, more than 4 million newborns die within the first days or weeks of life, and altogether 10.6 million children die each year before their fifth birthday. According to the 2009 World Health Organization (WHO) report, maternal and infant mortality is still among the worst performing health indicator in resource-poor countries and regions, and it has barely changed since 1990 (Say, Souza, and Patterson 2009, World Health Organization 2009). About 95 percent of the maternal deaths and 90 percent of the new-born deaths have occurred in developing countries (United Nations Children's Fund 2009), and most of these deaths are preventable (Save the Children Fund 2006). In addition, more than one quarter of all adult women living in developing countries currently suffer from short- or long-term illnesses and injuries related to pregnancy and childbirths (United Nations Children's Fund 2009). Given the current conditions in some developing countries, particularly the neglect of many of women's health needs and the assignment of their primary responsibilities in childrearing, improvement in maternal-child care appears to be a natural home for the improvement of women's reproductive health.

Third, the women's human rights hypothesis is not supported by the data from the 137 developing countries. The relationship between women's human rights and reproductive health is not statistically significant. The claim that reproductive health can be promoted through binding human rights instruments and treaties is not supported by the data used in the study. It is perhaps that human rights instruments provide a legal discourse for political functions and social welfare issues, but that the legal approach does not necessarily provide a moral and social foundation to ensure the implementation of social welfare and human well-being on the part of women, especially in developing countries (Ahmed-Ghosh 2006). Therefore, a formal legal approach may not be sufficient to achieve women's reproductive health as measured in this study. This finding indicates certain inconsistencies in the claim made by international conferences and conventions. This finding suggests that human rights legislations and instruments alone may not necessarily lead to the improvement of women's reproductive health.

The fourth finding indicates the importance of economic development in predicting maternal-child care. The direct path from economic development to maternal-child care is statistically significant ($p<.01$). As Caldwell (2001) proposed, economic development is closely associated with the shifts in health care and the most profound changes during the epidemiological transition are more likely to affect women and children. Numerous studies have found that breakthroughs in medical science and social changes as a result of economic development are important determinants of the improvement in health outcomes especially for women and children (Omran 1971, 1982, Bell 2001).

Finally, a positive and statistically significant relationship is found between economic development and gender equality. A study on the decline in infant mortality in India by Claeson , Bos, Mawji and Pathmanathan (2000) found that reproductive health can be improved without significant economic development. The finding from this study indicates otherwise. As I mentioned in Chapter 2, the relationship between economic development and gender equality has been a debated issue among social scientists and the empirical findings are inconsistent. Criticisms on the neoclassical economic theory evolve around its apolitical nature and a linear understanding of the relationship between economic development and gender equality. Peterson's (2003) analysis on the global economic models of reproductive, productive, and virtual economies challenged the gender-neutral assumptions of development and pointed to the exploitation of women's labor in reproduction and informal economy. The finding from the 137 developing countries, however, indicates that economic development is important in predicting gender equality. Economic growth, perhaps as a form of liberal ideology and technological advancement, can serve to redress gender equality in developing countries as a whole. Economic development may lead to changes in gender role expectations and government policies that work in favor of women's education, participation in the labor force and their involvement in political decision making (Zhang and Thomas 1994, Tay and Gibbons 1998). The finding from the 137 developing countries supports the hypothesis that economic development tends to lead to an increase in gender equality.

In sum, the proposed model of women's reproductive health is partially supported by the data from the 137 developing countries.

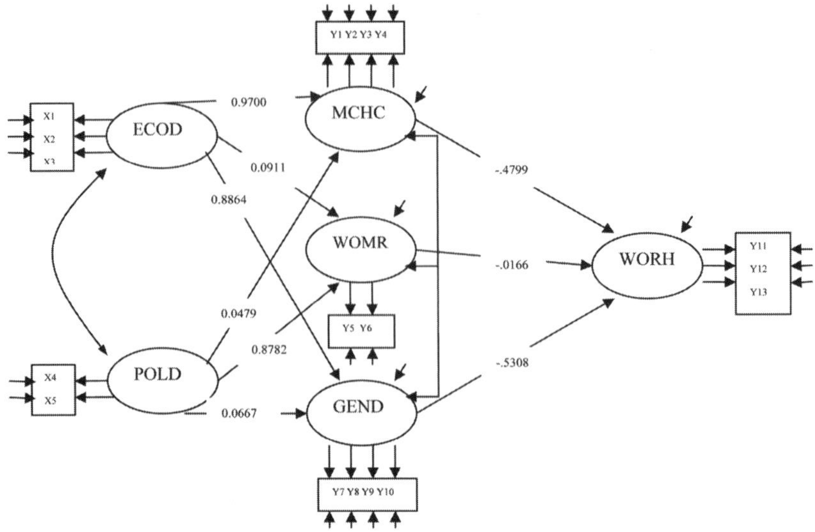

ECOD: Economic Development	X1: % population using adequate sanitation facilities X2: % population using safe water X3: % urban
POLD: Political Development	X4: political terror scale X5: Political freedom and civil liberty
MCHC: Maternal-Child Care	Y1: Skilled attendance at delivery Y2: Antenatal care coverage Y3: Children immunized against measles Y4: Contraceptive prevalence
WOMR: Women's Human Rights	Y5: Abortion right Y6: Women's economic, political, and social rights
GEND: Gender Equality	Y7: Female gross secondary enrollment Y8: Estimated female income Y9: Gender equity index Y10: Seats in parliament held by women
WORH: Women's Reproductive Health	Y11: Infant mortality Y12: Maternal mortality Y13: Infant with low birth weight

Figure 4.1 The Findings of the Structural Model

4.4 Alternative Model

The findings from the proposed model underscore the importance of gender equality and maternal-child care to predict women's reproductive health. As the empirical test of the proposed model has yielded partial support, the next step is to test a model that may yield a better fit to the data. The alternative model is evaluated using structural equation modeling. Table 4.5 presents the findings from the alternative structural model.

LISREL provides fit statistics about the adequacy of model fit. The results suggest that the alternative model has provided a much better fit to the data (GFI = 0.923; AGFI = 0.855). Note that GFI and AGFI measures are not affected by sample size and are robust against the departure from normality (Lavee 1988). A value closer to 1 indicates a better fit model. A small difference of less than 0.05 between GFI and AGFI indicates that the model fits well to the data. (As this study intends to test the theoretical explanations, the focus is on the estimation of the structural parameters of the model rather than achieving a best fit model.) A structural model with hypothesized linear relations is an approximation. It is unreasonable to expect a perfect model fit. In structural equation analysis, one can expect that the model fits well enough to be a reasonable explanation of the trends in the data (Bollen 1989, Maruyama 1997).

The findings indicate that both gender equality and maternal-child care are significant predictors of women's reproductive health. The direct effect of maternal-child care on women's reproductive health is strong and statistically

Table 4.5 Alternative Structural Model, LISREL Estimates (standardized estimates in parentheses)

Endogenous Factors	**Exogenous Factors**		
	ECOD	MCHC	GEND
MCHC	0.9575** (0.9932)	-----	-----
GEND	0.9534** (0.9228)	-----	-----
WORH	----- (-.7598)	-.7750** (-.2515)	-.2186**

GFI=0.923
AGFI=0.855
RMSR=0.044
Total coefficient of determination for structural equation =0.987

**: p<0.01
+: The negative sign "-" indicates that an increase in MCHC and GEND leads to an improvement in women's reproductive health. The discussion on the coding of women's reproductive health indicators can be found in Chapter 3.

significant (-0.7750). Gender equality is found to have a significant and moderate effect on women's reproductive health (-0.2186). The findings from the alternative structural model are presented in Figure 4.2.

A second most frequently used measure to assess model fit is the likelihood-ratio chi-square statistics (Joreskog and Sorbom 1989). Chi-square tests are used to determine whether the differences between the predicted variance-covariance matrix and the actual variance-covariance matrix approach zero. A statistically significant chi-square indicates a statistically significant discrepancy between the

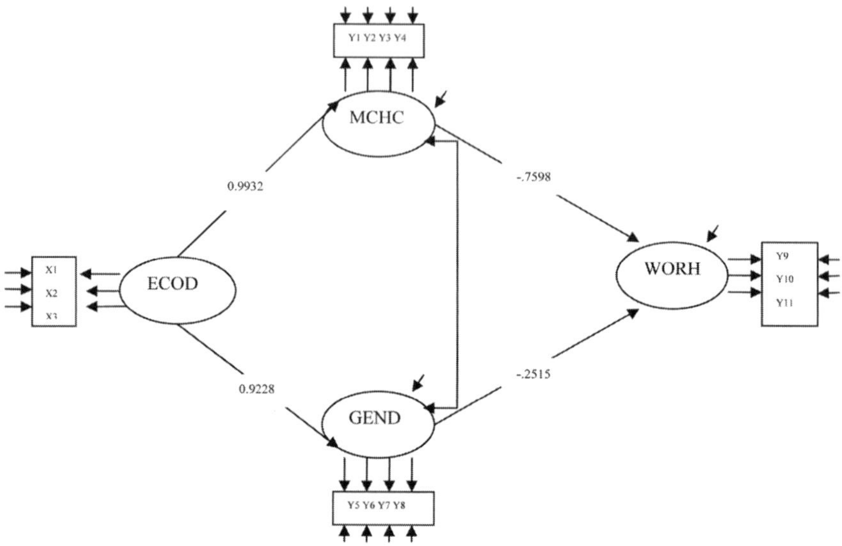

ECOD: Economic Development	X1: % population using adequate sanitation facilities X2: % population using safe water X3: % urban
MCHC: Maternal-Child Care	Y1: Skilled attendance at delivery Y2: Antenatal care coverage Y3: Children immunized against measles Y4: Contraceptive prevalence
GEND: Gender Equality	Y5: Female gross secondary enrollment Y6: Estimated female income Y7: Gender equity index Y8: Seats in parliament held by women
WORH: Women's Reproductive Health:	Y9: Infant mortality Y10: Maternal mortality Y11: Infant with low birth weight

Figure 4.2 Alternative Model

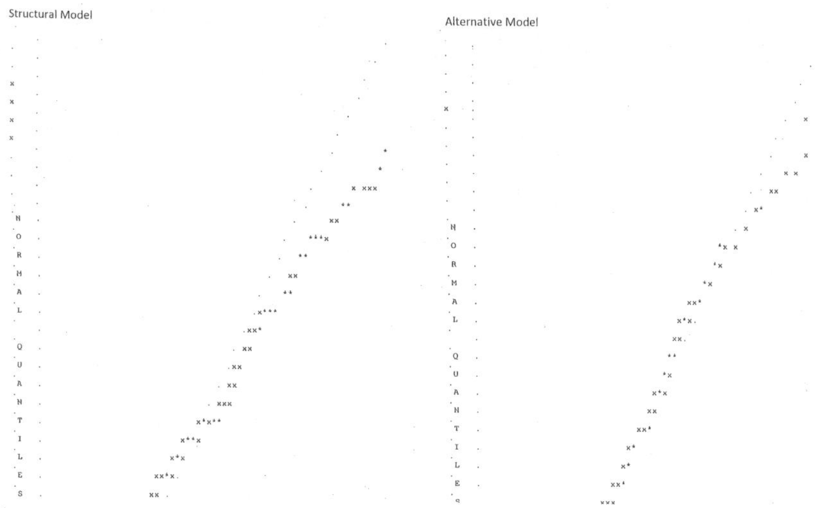

Figure 4.3 Q-Plot Comparison: Structural Model and Alternative Model

data and the model. When the hypothesized model perfectly fits the data, chi-square is small in relation to the degrees of freedom (df). A chi-square measure that is statistically insignificant indicates a good fit of the model to the data. In the case of the alternative model, chi-square = 70.67 (p = .090); df = 56. When a chi-square and df ratio is less than 5, it is often regarded as an indication of model fit.

Lavee (1998) cautioned against the use of chi-square statistics alone to assess model fit. Chi-square statistics assumes multivariate normality, which is difficult to assess. The model is more likely to be "fit" when the sample size is small. With these limitations in mind, Joreskog and Sorborn (1989) suggested the use of Q plot. Q-plot is a graph of the normalized residuals. When the residuals from the estimated model deviate away from the diagonal of the Q-plot graph, it suggests that the model is incorrectly specified. A comparison of the Q-plots of the proposed and alternative structural models is presented in Figure 4.3.

The residuals of the alternative structural model appear to be distributed more along the diagonal of the Q-plot graph. In summary, the alternative model yields a better fit to the data.

Chapter 5
Regional Variations

Sarah Curtis (2004), in the book titled *Health and Inequality: Geographical Perspectives*, stated that the geography of health is primarily concerned with the question of health variations in populations in different parts of the world and how we understand these variations. Beginning in the 1950s, regional science as a field of geography started to provide a strong quantitative base for human activity research in different regions. Findings, however, have been inconsistent. Ellaway and Mackintyre (1996), Gould and Jones (1996), and Shouls, Congdon, and Curtis (1996) found that areas of residence are related to the health conditions of the population independent of the characteristics of individuals, while Slogett and Joshi (1998) found no or little impact of the area or region variables on people's health.

Recent development in theories and empirical research on regional variations in health includes spatial epidemiology (Elliott and Wartenberg 2004), human geography (Harvey 2000), and economic geography (Huntington 2001), all of which are concerned with the analysis of geographic variations in illnesses and diseases with respect to demographic, environmental, and social-economic factors. In examining the variations in the health condition of a population in different places and the factors that contribute to regional variations in health, McKeown (1979, 1991), for instance, concluded that the health of a population is determined by the levels of social and economic development of the region. Berkman and Kawachi (2000) recognized that social structures and economic processes of the region are important to explain the health outcomes in different places. Curtis (2004) emphasized the link between the health condition of a population and the social and economic environment of the regions. In a 2003 publication, Fitzpatrick and LaGory used metropolitan regions as the units of analysis and linked the health risks of the population to the distinct spatial qualities of the cities. Fitzpatrick and LaGory (2003) called the analysis the "ecology of metropolitan regions."

To examine regional variations and the effects of region variables on women's reproductive health, this chapter contains four sections. The first section discusses the variations of women's reproductive health indicators across and within regions. Section two focuses on cluster analysis which is used to group countries (areas) with similar values on women's reproductive health scores. Section three provides discussions on the tests of the statistical significance in regional variations. Section four discusses the dilemma of the sub-Saharan Africa region with regard to women's reproductive health conditions.

The 137 developing countries (or areas) are divided into six regions: sub-Saharan Africa (N=45), Arab states (N=20), East Asia/Pacific (N=28), South Asia (N=9), Latin America/Caribbean (N=33), and Southern Europe (N=2) (Appendix

E. Developing Countries in Regional Aggregates).[1] As Southern Europe consists of only two countries, the region is not included in the regional analysis in the third section.

5.1 Regional Variations in Women's Reproductive Health Indicators

I. Maternal Mortality

Complications during pregnancy and childbirth are the leading cause of deaths and disability among women of reproductive age in developing countries (United Nations Children's Fund 2004, United Nations Fund for Population Activities 2009, World Health Organization 2009). Women in sub-Saharan Africa face the highest risk in pregnancy- and childbirth-related deaths compared with women in the other regions of developing countries. On average, there are 821 maternal deaths per 100,000 live births in the sub-Saharan continent. South Asia has the second highest rate, close to 529 maternal deaths per 100,000 live births. Southern Europe has the lowest maternal mortality rate, about 58.5 per 100,000 live births. Of the other three regions, Latin America/Caribbean has the lowest maternal mortality rate, about 150 maternal deaths per 100,000 live births. Maternal mortality rate on average is slightly lower in the East Asia/Pacific region (182.77 per 100,000 live births) compared with Arab states (236.85 per 100,000 live births). Table 5.1 presents the regional variations in maternal mortality.

Within the sub-continent, there are considerable differences in maternal mortality rates. Seventeen out of the 45 countries (37.8 percent) in the region have maternal mortality rates 1,000 or higher per 100,000 live births according to the data from the United Nations Children's Fund (UNICEF 2008). These countries are: Sierra Leone (2,000), Malawi (1,800), Angola (1,700), Niger

Table 5.1 Regional Variations: Maternal Mortality (per 100,000 live births)

Region	Mean	Median	Minimum	Maximum
sub-Saharan Africa (N=45)	821.1333	800,0000	24	2,000
Arab States (N=20)	236.8500	130.0000	5	1,100
East Asia/Pacific (N=22)	182.7727	125.0000	20	660
South Asia (N=9)	528.6667	420.0000	76	1,900
Latin America/Caribbean (N=33)	149.9091	110.000	1	680
South Europe (N=2)	58.5000	58.5000	47	70

1 The classification of developing countries can be found in the United Nations' *Human Development Report 2007–2008*. http://hdr.undp.org/en/media/HDR_20072008_en_complete.pdf.

(1,600), Tanzania United Rep. (1,500), Rwanda (1,400), Mali (1,200), Central African Rep. (1,100), Chad (1,100), Guinea Bissau (1,100), Zimbabwe (1,100), Burundi (1,000), Eritrea (1,000), Kenya (1,000), Burkina Faso (1,000), Mauritania (1,000), and Mozambique (1,000). Mauritius (24) and Seychelles (57) have the lowest maternal mortality rates. (As far as the mortality data are concerned, it is sometimes difficult to trace and measure maternal mortality trends in a number of African countries mainly because of the lack of vital registration systems to monitor the trends in spite of the fact that tens of thousands of African women are killed every year due to pregnancy and childbirth.)

II. Infant Mortality

Sub-Saharan Africa remains the highest infant mortality rate in the world. On average, of 100 babies born alive in sub-Saharan Africa, nine will die before reaching their first birthday (91.73 per 1,000 live births) according to the data from the United Nations Children's Fund (UNICEF 2008). The South Asia region is the second highest, 61.22 per 1,000 live births. The lowest infant mortality rates occur in Latin America/Caribbean (22.45 per 1,000 live births) and South Europe (15 per 1,000 live births). Infant mortality rate is slightly higher for Arab states (37.8 per 1,000 live births) than for East Asia/Pacific (32.3 per 1,000 live births). Table 5.2 presents the regional variations in infant mortality.

Of all of the sub-Saharan African countries, Sierra Leone has the highest infant mortality rate, 165 per 1,000 live births, whereas Mauritius (13 per 1,000 live births) and Seychelles (12 per 1,000 live births) have the lowest infant mortality rates. About 42 percent (19 countries) of the countries in sub-Saharan Africa have infant mortality rates 100 or above per 1,000 live births. These countries are: Sierra Leone (165), Liberia (157), Angola (154), Niger (150), Congo D. (Zaire) (129), Chad (124), Guinea Bissau (124), Equatorial Guinea (123), Mali (120), Cote d'Ivoire (118), Rwanda (118), Central African Rep. (115), Burundi (114), Swaziland (110), Ethiopia (109), Lesotho (102), Zambia (102), Mozambique (100), and Nigeria (100).

Table 5.2 Regional Variations: Infant Mortality (per 1,000 live births)

Region	Mean	Median	Minimum	Maximum
sub-Saharan Africa (N=45)	91.7333	89.0000	12	165
Arab States (N=20)	37.8000	21.5000	8	133
East Asia/Pacific (N=27)	32.3333	25.0000	3	98
South Asia (N=9)	61.2222	56.0000	12	165
Latin America/Caribbean (N=33)	22.4545	18.0000	6	84
South Europe (N=2)	15.0000	15.0000	2	26

III. Infants with Low Birth Weight (infants who weigh less than 2,500 grams)

According to the data from the United Nations Children's Fund (UNICEF 2008), about one in five infants is under weight for age in South Asia (21.5 percent), followed by sub-Saharan Africa (15.17 percent), Arab states (12.32 percent), Latin America/Caribbean (12.21 percent), and East Asia/Pacific (9.27 percent). Table 5.3 presents the regional variations in the percentage of infants with low birth weight.

Table 5.3 Regional Variations: Percentage Infants with Low Birth Weight (less than 2,500 grams)

Region	Mean	Median	Minimum	Maximum
sub-Saharan Africa (N=41)	15.1707	14.0000	9	25
Arab States (N=19)	12.3158	10.0000	6	32
East Asia/Pacific (N=26)	9.2692	9.0000	0	20
South Asia (N=8)	21.5000	21.5000	7	36
Latin America/Caribbean (N=33)	10.2121	9.0000	5	23
South Europe (N=1)	16.0000	16.0000	16	16

The largest within region differences between the highest and lowest percentages are found in the South Asia and Arab states regions, followed by East Asia/Pacific, Latin America/Caribbean, and sub-Saharan Africa. About one third of the infants are under weight in Bangladesh (36 percent), India (30 percent), Sudan (31 percent), and Yemen (32 percent).

A comparison of the regional variations in women's reproductive health indicators is presented in Figure 5.1. The highest maternal and infant mortality rates are found in the sub-Saharan Africa region, while the South Asia region leads in the percentage of infants with low birth weight.

5.2 Cluster Analysis

Cluster analysis is a method for grouping items to assess similarities based on the occurrence or non-occurrence of particular characteristics. In other words, cluster analysis is a process of grouping data in ways where the degree of association is strong between members of the same cluster and weak between members of different clusters. Table 5.4 presents the clusters of nations in terms of women's

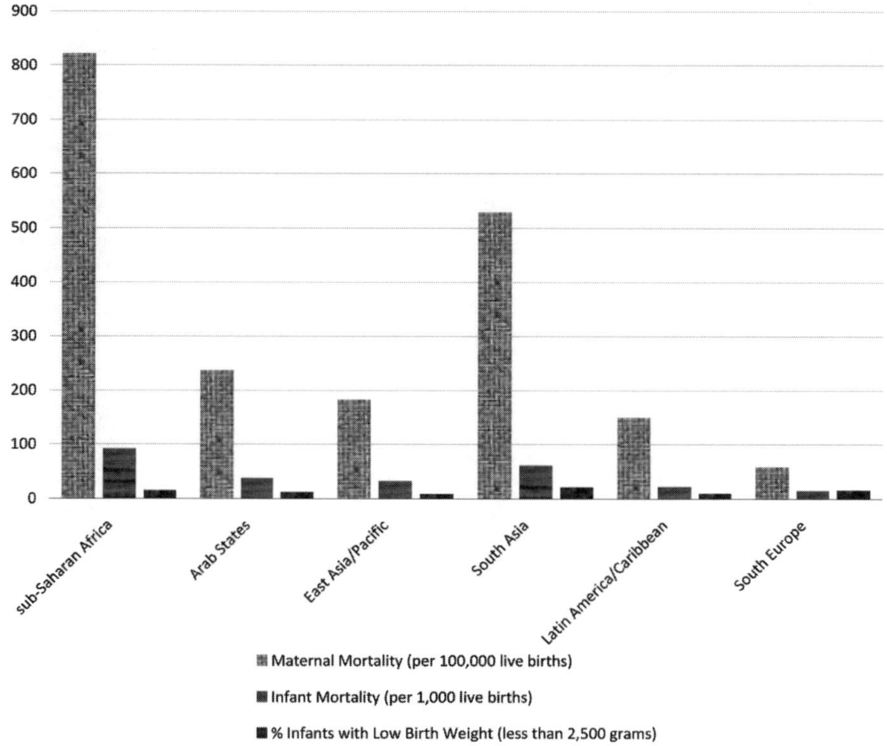

Figure 5.1 Comparison of Regional Variations

reproductive health by using the nearest neighbor method. Of the 137 developing countries, seven clusters are formed using the nearest neighboring approach.[2]

The assignment of women's reproductive health score for each country is obtained by using exploratory factor analysis of the three indicators. Seven clusters are formed at the fourth stage. Clusters 2, 3, 6, and 7 consist of most sub-Saharan African countries and two other countries, one from South Asia (Bangladesh) and the other from the Arab region (Yemen). Only seven countries fall into clusters 2, 6, and 7. These seven countries that are separated from most developing countries are among the least developed countries in the world. Table 5.5 presents the social and economic characteristics of the seven countries in comparison with all developing countries and the world.

On the contrary, of the 62 countries in cluster 1, only two countries are in the sub-Saharan Africa region, Cape Verde and Mauritius. About half of the

2 Of the 137 developing countries, 13 countries are excluded (9.5 percent) due to missing data for one or more variables of the three indicators of women's reproductive health.

Table 5.4 Cluster Analysis: Women's Reproductive Health

Cluster	Country (Area)	Cluster	Country (Area)	Cluster	Country (Area)
1	Algeria (AR)	2	Angola (AF)	3	Bangladesh (SA)
	Antigua Barbuda (LA)		Niger (AF)		Burkina Faso (AF)
	Argentina (LA)				Burundi (AF)
	Bahamas (LA)	4	Benin (AF)		Central African Rep (AF)
	Bahrain (AR)		Bhutan (SA)		Congo (D) (AF)
	Barbados (LA)		Botswana (AF)		Cote d'Ivoire AF)
	Belize (LA)		Cambodia (EA)		Equatorial Guinea (AF)
	Brazil (LA)		Cameroon (AF)		Ethiopia (AF)
	Brunei Darussalam (EA)		Comoros (AF)		Mozambique (AF)
	Cape Verde (AF)		Djibouti (AR)		Rwanda (AF)
	Chile (LA)		Eritrea (AF)		Sudan (AR)
	China (EA)		Gabon (AF)		Tanzania (AF)
	Colombia (LA)		Gambia (AF)		Yemen (AR)
	Costa Rica (LA)		Ghana (AF)		
	Cuba (LA)		Guinea (AF)	5	Bolivia (LA)
	Dominica (LA)		Haiti (LA)		Guyana (LA)
	Dominican Rep. (LA)		India (SA)		Maldives (SA)
	Ecuador (LA)		Iraq (AR)		Micronesia (EA)
	Egypt (AR)		Kenya (AF)		Morocco (AR)
	El Salvador (LA)		Laos (EA)		Namibia (AF)
	Fiji (EA)		Lesotho (AF)		Papua New Guinea (EA)
	Grenada (LA)		Madagascar (AF)		Philippines (EA)
	Guatemala (LA)		Myanmar (EA)		South Africa (AF)
	Honduras (LA)		Nepal (SA)		Sri Lanka (SA)
	Indonesia (EA)		Nigeria(AF)		Trinidad & Tobago (LA)
	Iran (SA)		Pakistan (SA)		
	Jamaica (LA)		Sao Tome & Principe (AF)	6	Chad (AF)
	Jordan (AR)		Senegal (AF)		Guinea-Bissau (AF)
	Kiribati (EA)		Swaziland (AF)		Malawi (AF)
	Korea (D) (EA)		Timor-Leste (EA)		Mali (AF)
	Korea (R) (EA)		Togo (AF)		
	Kuwait (AR)		Uganda (AF)	7	Sierra Leone (AF)
	Lebanon (AR)		Zambia (AF)		
	Libyan Arab Jamahiriya (AR)		Zimbabwe (AF)		
	Malaysia (EA)				
	Mauritius (AF)				
	Mexico (LA)				
	Mongolia (EA)				
	Nicaragua (LA)				
	Occupied Palestinian Territory (AR)				
	Oman (AR)				
	Panama (LA)				
	Paraguay (LA)				

Cluster	Country (Area)	Cluster	Country (Area)	Cluster	Country (Area)
	Peru (LA)				
	Qatar (AR)				
	St. Kitts & Nevis (LA)				
	St. Lucia (LA)				
	St. Vincent & Grenadines (LA)				
	Samoa (EA)				
	Saudi Arabia (AR)				
	Singapore (EA)				
	Solomon Islands (EA)				
	Suriname (LA)				
	Syrian Arab Rep (AR)				
	Thailand (EA)				
	Tunisia (AR)				
	Turkey (SE)				
	United Arab Emirates (AR)				
	Uruguay (LA)				
	Vanuatu (EA)				
	Venezuela (LA)				
	Vietnam (EA)				

AF: sub-Saharan Africa; AR: Arab states; EA: East Asia/Pacific; SA: South Asia; LA: Latin America/Caribbean; SE: South Europe.

Table 5.5 Selected Social and Economic Characteristics of the Least Developed Countries

Country	Human Development Index (HDI)	Life Expectancy in years	Adult Literacy %	Urban Population %	GDP per capita $
Angola	0.446	41.7	67.4	53.3	2,335
Chad	0.388	50.4	25.7	25.3	1,427
Guinea Bissau	0.374	45.8		29.6	827
Malawi	0.437	46.3	64.1	17.2	667
Mali	0.380	53.1	24.0	30.5	1,033
Niger	0.374	55.8	28.7	16.8	781
Sierra Leone	0.336	41.8	34.8	40.7	806
All developing countries	0.691	66.1	76.7	42.7	5,282
High-income OECD	0.947	79.4		77.0	33,831
World	0.743	68.1	78.6	48.6	9,453

Source: United Nations Development Programme (UNDP). 2008. *Human Development Report 2007–2008*.

countries in this cluster are in the Latin-American/Caribbean region. None of the countries in the Latin America/Caribbean region is found in cluster 4 except for Haiti. Eleven countries fall into cluster 5. Three countries are in Latin America/ Caribbean (Bolivia, Guyana, and Trinidad & Tobago); two countries are in South Asia (Maldives, Sri Lanka), three countries are in East Asia/Pacific (Micronesia, Papua New Guinea, and the Philippines), two countries are in sub-Saharan Africa (Namibia, South Africa), and one country is in the Arab region (Morocco).

The results from the cluster analysis indicate that the sub-Saharan African region deviates from the other regions and continues to face more serious challenges than the other regions of developing countries with regard to the conditions of women's reproductive health and the reduction of maternal and infant mortality. Discussions on the impact of the region variables on women's reproductive health are presented in the next section.

5.3 OLS Estimates of Regional Variations

To test the strength of the region variables on women's reproductive health, multiple regression analysis is used. It is probably the most widely used statistical technique in the social sciences to estimate the magnitude of the impact of independent variables on dependent variable. Table 5.6 presents the estimates from

Table 5.6 OLS Estimates of the Effects of Regional Variables on Women's Reproductive Health

Variable	Equation 1		Equation 2	
	b	Beta	b	Beta
Arab States	-1.419***	-.513	-.773***	-.263
East Asia/Pacific	-1.550***	-.595	-.889***	-.258
South Asia	-0.612*	-.151	-.449*	-.108
Latin American/ Caribbean	-1.682***	-.746	-.735***	-.318
Maternal-Child Care			-.465***	-.443
Gender Equality			-.266***	-.238
R^2	0.557		0.835	
Adjusted R^2	0.542		0.823	
(Constant)	0.980***		0.541***	

*: $p<0.05$
***: $p<0.001$

two different regression equations. For both equations, the dependent variable is the factor score of women reproductive health indicators.

Equation 1 contains four dummy region variables. The reference category for the region dummies is sub-Saharan Africa. Ordinary Least Square (OLS) analysis is used for the cross-sectional data. The assumption for the OLS model is that target data are randomly sampled from a population and are independent of each other (Allison 1999, Pickett, Reilly, and McIntyre 2005). The "b" column contains the regression coefficients and the "Beta" column contains the standardized coefficients. All of the regions in Equation 1 (Arab state, East Asia/Pacific, South Asia, and Latin America/Caribbean) are significantly different from sub-Saharan Africa in women's reproductive health scores. Of the four regions, Latin America/Caribbean appears to hold the largest gap from sub-Saharan Africa, followed by East Asia/Pacific and Arab states (***: $p<.001$). As shown at the bottom of Table 5.6, the single asterisk for the South Asia region indicates a coefficient whose "p" value is less than .05. It means if the South Asia region variable had no effect, the probability of finding a coefficient as large as or larger than the least squares estimate is less than five in a hundred. For Equation 1, the R^2 is .557, which means that about 56 percent of the variation in women's reproductive health scores can be explained by the four region variables.

The next question is how much of the association between the region variables and women's reproductive health scores can be explained by their relationships with other variables. Equation 2 adds two more variables, maternal-child care and gender equality. By comparing the coefficients for region variables in both equations, we can see that the effect of the region variables on women's reproductive health does not change with the controls. The four regions are still significantly different from sub-Saharan Africa with regard to women's reproductive health. But the coefficients of the region variables in Equation 2 are cut almost in half, which tells us that the maternal-child care and gender equality variables have played an important role in mediating the impact of the region variables on women's reproductive health. The R^2 for Equation 2 rises to 0.835, meaning that the region variables together with the two controls can explain almost 84 percent of the variation in women's reproductive health.

The findings from the multiple regression analysis indicate that sub-Saharan African countries, as a whole, are facing major challenges to reduce pregnancy related deaths and to improve women's reproductive health in comparison with Latin America/Caribbean, East Asia/Pacific, Arab states, and South Asia. The challenges to improve the reproductive health of millions of African women are more daunting than those in other regions.

5.4 The sub-Saharan Africa Dilemma

Based on the findings from the 137 developing countries, the situation of women's reproductive health is most dire in sub-Saharan Africa compared with the other regions under study.

Maternal mortality is one of the reproductive health indicators that underscores the largest gap between sub-Saharan Africa and other regions and countries in the world. While there were only nine maternal deaths per 100,000 live deaths in developed countries as a whole in 2005, there were 450 maternal deaths per 100,000 live births in developing countries (Glasier, Gulmezoglu, Schmid, Moreno, and Look 2006, United Nations 2009). The sub-Saharan Africa region is found to have the highest maternal mortality rates. In sub-Saharan Africa, maternal deaths can be as high as more than 1,000 per 100,000 live births in some of its countries. In 2007, over 99 percent of the maternal deaths in the world occurred in developing countries and half of all of these maternal deaths occurred in sub-Saharan Africa (and another third occurred in South Asia). Together, these two regions accounted for 85 percent of all maternal deaths during that year (United Nations 2009). According to the United Nations Fund for Population Activities (UNFPA) and the Population Research Bureau (PRB) (2005) and the United Nations Children Fund (UNICEF), the World Health Organization (WHO), and the United Nations Fund for Population Activities (UNFPA) (2007), women in sub-Saharan Africa face an average of 1 in 16 lifetime risk of dying from pregnancy related causes, compared to 1 in 7,300 for women in developed countries.

With regard to infant and child mortality, a recent survey found that infant and child morality has increased in some sub-Saharan African countries, while infant and child survival rates have improved by nearly 30 percent in surveyed developing countries since 1990. For example, in the year 2000, 43 percent of child deaths in the world were among children living in sub-Saharan Africa compared with 14 percent in 1960. According to a 2009 report of the United Nations, child mortality rate has declined steadily worldwide, and the global under-five mortality rate in 2007 stayed at 67 deaths per 1,000 live births. For developing countries as a whole, under-five mortality rate was 74 per 1,000 live births during the year 2007. In sub-Saharan Africa, however, in 2007, close to one in seven children died before their fifth birthday, from 4.2 million in 1990 to 4.6 million in 2007. Sub-Saharan Africa now accounts for half of all of the deaths among children under five, a seven percent increase compared with the year 2000.

Sub-Saharan Africa continues to suffer disproportionally from the HIV/AIDS epidemic. There are four striking features of the HIV/AIDS epidemic in the sub-Saharan Africa region. The first feature is the "feminization" of the disease and the disproportionate burden of the virus on women. Worldwide, women represent nearly half of the 40 million HIV-positive individuals. In sub-Saharan Africa, however, 57 percent of the adults with HIV are women, and women aged 15 to 24 are more than three times as likely to be infected as men of the same age group (United Nations Fund for Population Activities 2004a). Two-thirds of those newly infected with HIV in sub-Saharan Africa are women and girls (United Nations Joint Programme on HIV/AIDS 2006). According to the United Nations (2009), an estimated 15 million children worldwide had lost one or both parents to AIDS by the end of 2007; and about 12 million of them (80 percent) lived in sub-Saharan Africa. In addition, an estimated 47.5 million children in the Sub-Saharan Africa region had lost one or both parents to AIDS or other causes as of 2007 (United Nation 2009).

Second, the disease spreads throughout the general population rather than being confined to the population at risk, such as injecting drug users, sex workers and their clients, and men who have sex with other men. Third, there are considerable variations within the region in terms of the percentages of people living with HIV/AIDS, from 38.8 percent to 0.1 percent. Southern Africa is home to the fasted growing epidemic in the world. Botswana leads the whole Southern African area with a HIV/AIDS prevalence rate of 38.8 percent. The second highest is Swaziland, where 38.6 percent of the Swazi have been infected with HIV/AIDS. The other Southern African countries with HIV/AIDS prevalence rate above 15 percent are Zimbabwe (33.7 percent), Lesotho (31 percent), Namibia (22.5 percent), Zambia (21.5 percent), South Africa (20.1 percent), and Malawi (15.1 percent). Kenya in Eastern Africa has a prevalence rate of 15 percent. The lowest rate is 0.1 percent for Mauritius. According to the United Nations Economic and Social Affairs (UNESA 2006), of the 62 countries in the world that are considered to be highly affected by the HIV/AIDS epidemic, 40 of them are located in sub-Saharan Africa. (Note that there are 45 countries in the sub-Saharan Africa region.) The fourth feature is the increase in the number of new infections that has occurred each year since 2000. Although the percentage of people living with HIV/AIDS in the region has leveled off since 2000, the total number has steadily increased largely due to new infections that still outnumber AIDS deaths.

The challenges to reduce maternal and infant mortality and to improve women's reproductive health in sub-Saharan Africa were further compounded by the economic fabric that has deteriorated in recent decades due to wars and other human inflicted occurrences. Massive human displacements in the wake of armed conflicts and natural disasters have taken a huge toll on civilians in the countries of sub-Saharan Africa. Worldwide, by the end of 2008, there were about 15 million refugees and 26 million internationally displaced persons (IDPs) (United Nations High Commissioner for Refugees 2008). According to the United Nations High Commissioner for Refugees (UNHCR 2008) and Bonn International Center for Conversion (BICC 2009), over 2.1 million refugees and about 12.7 million internally displaced persons had lived in Africa by the end of 2008.[3] Of those refugees and internally displaced persons, about

3 According to the United Nations High Commissioner for Refugees (2008), Afghanistan has been the leading country of origin of refugees for the past three decades. By the end of 2008, there were more than 2.8 million Afghan refugees.

80 percent are women and children (Women's Commission for Refugee Women and Children 2006, United Nations High Commissioner for Refugees 2008, Bonn International Center for Conversion 2009); of these women and children, about 20 percent are of reproductive age and 25 percent of them are expectant mothers (Centers for Disease Control and Prevention 2006b, Women's Commission for Refugee Women and Children 2006, United Nations High Commissioner for Refugees 2008, Bonn International Center for Conversion 2009). In addition, there is an unknown number of women of reproductive age who are internally displaced and homeless due to natural disasters and construction projects (Esscher 2004, United Nations High Commissioner for Refugees – 2008). These people are forced to live in an environment of severe instability, where educational and health care systems have collapsed, HIV and other sexually transmitted infections have increased, and infant and maternal mortality rates have skyrocketed (United Nations Fund for Populations Activities 2005, United Nations High Commissioner for Refugees 2008). According to the *State of the World's Mothers Report* (Save the Children 2002, 2003, 2009), of the ten countries that rank the lowest in Mother's Index due to war or some kind of conflicts, nine are in sub-Saharan Africa.[4] The nine countries are Benin, Gambia, Guinea, Ethiopia, Mali, Yemen, Guinea Bissau, Burkina Faso, and Niger. In addition, of the ten countries with the highest child mortality rates, seven are in the mist of or recovering from war or armed conflicts; and six of them are in the sub-Saharan Africa region.[5]

The harsh circumstances of war and armed conflicts can have disastrous and lasting impact on women and children. Prior to the mid-1990s, however, there was very little systematic research on women's reproductive health and pregnancy-related problems among refugees and internally displaced persons (Jamieson, Meikle, Hills, Mtsuko, Mawji, and Duerr 2000, Harris and Smyth 2001). And very little attention was given to the reproductive health needs of refugees and displaced persons in spite of the fact that reproductive health related problems are a major cause of morbidity and mortality among women and girls in war and armed conflicts. During the mid and late 1990s, several events contributed to the increasing recognition of the reproductive health needs among refugees and internally displaced persons (Krause, Jones, and Purdin 2000). In 1994, the Women's Commission for Refugee Women and Children (WCRWC) published an influential report documenting the lack of reproductive health services for refugees and internally displaced persons, particularly those in sub-Saharan Africa. The Inter-agency Working Group on Refugee Health (IAWG) was then formed,

4 Mother's Index developed by Save the Children (www.savethechildren.org) is a composite measure of two indices (women's index and children's index) based on ten indicators pertaining to the well-being of mothers and children, including lifetime risk of maternal mortality, infant mortality, and their nutritional status.

5 The six countries in sub-Saharan Africa are Angola, Democratic Republic of Congo, Liberia, Mozambique, Sierra Leone, and Somalia.

consisting of representatives of the United Nations agencies, governmental and non-governmental organizations (NGOs). IAWG produced a manual that identified specific areas and standards in refugee settings, such as minimum initial service package (MISP),[6] safe motherhood, sexual and gender-based violence, sexually transmitted diseases (STDs), family planning, and other reproductive health concerns. Around the same time, representatives of a group of NGOs joined together and formed the Reproductive Health for Refugees Consortium (RHRC) to increase refugees' access to reproductive health services. In 1995, the United Nations High Commissioner for Refugees (UNHCR), the United Nations Fund for Population Activities (UNFPA), the World Health Organization (WHO), and more than 50 United Nations governmental and non-governmental organizations met at a symposium for a global evaluation of reproductive health in conflict settings. The Symposium called for urgent international actions and systematic research on unwanted pregnancy and safe abortion, STDs, infant and maternal mortality, and gender-based violence among refugees and internally displaced persons in developing countries and sub-Saharan Africa in particular with a view to suggesting social policies and program effectiveness evaluations. In 1998, the International Rescue Committee (IRC), in collaboration with the United Nations Development Programme (UNDP) and the United Nations Development Fund for Women (UNIFEM) implemented the prevention and management of sexual violence component of the MISP in Congo-Brazzaville and they also provided intensive training to professionals on addressing the medical, psychological, and legal aspects of sexual violence within the reproductive health program (Krause, Jones, and Purdin 2000). At the same time, the Centers for Disease Control and Prevention's (CDC) Division of Reproductive Health (DRH) started a formal reproductive health in crises program for refugees and internally displaced persons in the emergency phase in post emergency camps and those who have returned to their countries of origin. (Appendix F. List of Selected Web Sites: Reproductive Health among Refugees and Internally Displaced Persons).

6 Minimum initial service package (MISP) is a minimum set of priority reproductive health activities to be put into motion during the earliest days of a refugee crisis. The purpose of which is to reduce short- and long-term reproductive health related morbidity and mortality. The package includes (1) identify an organization(s) and individual(s) to facilitate the coordination and implementation of the MISP; (2) prevent and manage the consequences of sexual violence; (3) reduce HIV transmission by enforcing respect for universal precautions against HIV/AIDS and by guaranteeing the availability of free condoms; (4) prevent excess neonatal and maternal morbidity and mortality by providing clean delivery kits for use by mothers or birth attendants to promote clean home deliveries, by providing midwife delivery kits to facilitate clean and safe deliveries at the health facilities, and by initiating the establishment of a referral system to manage obstetric emergencies; and (5) plan for the provision of comprehensive reproductive health services and integrate into Primary Health Care, as the situation permits (United Nations Fund for Population Activities 2000).

Since 2000, however, funding for refugee reproductive health programs has declined, largely due to the continuing perception at some level of the United Nations and certain world organizations that reproductive health is not an essential part or priority of an emergency response. A recent assessment conducted by United Nations Fund for Population Activities (UNFPA 2004b) in 2004 during the Sudanese refugee crisis in Chad found that most of the humanitarian workers were not familiar with the MISP (minimum initial service package) activities, and therefore did not efficiently implement the MISP. According to the United Nations High Commissioner for Refugees (UNHCR 2008), refugees, internally displaced persons, and others affected by emergencies, especially women of reproductive age in sub-Saharan Africa and some countries in south Asia, face multiple difficulties in accessing reproductive health care services.

Another factor that has contributed to the deteriorating economic fabric in sub-Saharan Africa is the change in the dynamics of the global economy. The current trend of globalization has caused greater health inequalities, particularly in women's reproductive health in sub-Saharan Africa, as a result of its concentration and flow of financial capital and persistent debt crises in developing countries (Schrecker, Labonte, and De Vogli 2008).

Globalization has presented itself with inconsistent realities and is having unprecedented impact on people's lives of every continent, especially women and children in sub-Saharan Africa. On the one hand, cross-border and trans-border flows of goods, services, investments and currencies between countries have spurred economic growth in some countries. On the other hand, the international division of labor has led to intensified competitions on a global labor market where employers compete for highly skilled labor force in developing countries to maximize their financial returns and, at the same time, low-income countries contend for foreign investments and contract production. Accordingly, as the World Bank (2009) predicted in its 2009 *World Development Report*, between-country economic and health inequalities have increased in many of the developing countries, especially countries in sub-Saharan Africa where the "unskilled population" is abundant and maternal and infant mortality rates are by far the highest. Goesling and Firebaugh (2004) and Cornia, Rosignoli, and Tiberti (2007), pointed out that between-country health inequalities increased from 1992 to 2000 in a significant reversal of the long-term trend. McMichael, McKee, Skolnikov, and Valkonen (2004) identified 42 countries, mostly in Sub-Saharan Africa, that had lower life expectancy from birth in the most recent years than in 1960, 1980, or 1990 largely due to increases in AIDS epidemic and infant and maternal mortality. Goesling and Firebaugh (2004) further pointed out that "Sub-Saharan Africa is central to the story of between-country health inequality in the late 20th century" (p. 140), in spite of the fact that only one-tenth of the world's population live there. Data have shown that the divergence in health inequality indicators, particularly infant and maternal mortality, will disappear if sub-Saharan Africa is removed from the sample (Schrecker, Labonte, and De Vogli 2008, World Bank 2009).

Sub-Saharan Africa is the poorest region in the world. According to the World Bank report (2009), for 2005, there were 1.4 billion people in developing countries (one quarter of the population) who lived on $1.25 or less per day in 2005 prices. While "poverty rate in East Asia fell from 80 percent" in the 1980s to "under 20 percent over this period," the sub-Saharan Africa region "stayed at around 50 percent…" (Cited from Chen and Ravallion 2008, policy research paper 4703). Based on the United Nations 2009 Millennium Development Goals Report, sub-Saharan Africa counted 100 million more extremely poor people in 2005 than in 1990 and its poverty rate remained at 50 percent. "No progress at all is foreseen for the working poor in sub-Saharan Africa even under the best-case scenario." (United Nations 2009: 9). To make it even worse, over the past 30 years, sub-Saharan Africa's population has grown faster than that of any other regions of developing countries even with the AIDS epidemic that has reversed decades of gains in its life expectancy (United Nations Fund for Population Activities and Population Research Bureau 2003, United Nations Fund for Population Activities and Population Research Bureau 2005). The region's youth bulge and the high proportion of people aged 0–14 (41.4 percent in 2005) in combination with the high percentage of people living in poverty can imply that the population momentum will probably continue for decades to come and its population size may research about 1.1 billion by the year 2025 (United Nations Economic and Social Affairs – UNESA 2006).

The sub-Saharan Africa region is behind on many of the Millennium Development Goals (MDGs) and is especially deficient in the areas of women's reproductive health to "reduce child mortality" (MDGs, Goal 4), to "improve maternal health" (MDGs, Goal 5),[7] and to "combat HIV/AIDS, malaria and other diseases" (MDGs, Goal 6) (Gribble and Haffey 2008). Very little progress has been made in sub-Saharan Africa where women face the greatest lifetime risk of dying as a result of pregnancy and childbirth in spite of the progress that has been made in women's reproductive health in many of the developing countries. The challenges facing sub-Saharan Africa to decrease the percentage of people living in extreme poverty, improve gender equality and empower women, and to reduce maternal and infant mortality are more daunting than in any other regions in the developing world. The sub-Saharan Africa experience indicates that international actions aimed at improving the reproductive health conditions of millions of women in the developing world, especially those in sub-Saharan Africa have barely been effective, probably because the benefits of growth may rarely reach the poorest populations in the world (Woodward and Simms 2006, Schrecker, Labonte, and De Vogli 2008).

---

7 The Millennium Development Goals (MDGs) called for a three quarter reduction in maternal mortality between 1990 and 2015 (Goal 5, Target 5). It is very unlikely that most sub-Saharan African countries will have met this goal by the year 2015 (Gribble and Haffey 2008).

Given the vast across- and within-region disparities in women's reproductive health and the challenges facing sub-Saharan Africa, this study recommends that governments and the international community make extensive and strong commitments to prioritize and advance women's education, political participation, and financial independence and, further to reduce maternal and infant mortality and to improve women's reproductive health conditions in the sub-Saharan Africa region.

Chapter 6
Discussion and Implications

This chapter consists of four sections and provides thoughts and comments on the empirical findings from the proposed model. The first section, Enhancing Gender Equality Approach to Women's Reproductive Health, starts with a review of the historical background and moves on to the analysis of the gender equality approach to women's reproductive health. The second section focuses on the social policy issues. Section three provides comments on the limitations of the study and the need for more empirical research. The last section presents a brief summary of this study.

6.1 Enhancing Gender Equality Approach to Women's Reproductive Health

The issue of women's reproductive health and gender equality has become one of the core issues among social scientists and feminist scholars. Women's lack of access to education and other social, political, and economic resources have made them unable to protect their own health and the health of their children, especially women living in developing countries. Feminist scholars and social scientists are critical of the biomedical model that discounts the socially constructed constraints on women's health, such as social norms, traditions, codes, and practices. Keleher and Franklin (2008) stated that social norms and codes are embedded in the social structure and operated to restrict the opportunities and capacities of women and girls. In the early 1990s, Geoffrey Rose (1994) wrote, in the book titled *The Strategy of Preventive Medicine*, that the primary determinants of ill health and diseases, including women's reproductive health, are mainly economic and social and that remedies must also be economic and social. In the meantime, Rebecca Cook (1995) and Sen, George, and Östlin (2002) pointed out that medicine has evolved into a science dominated by biological revelations achieved in laboratories and hospitals and that health professionals have conscientiously looked for physiological and psychiatric causes of ill health. As a result, hospital-based medical practices have become isolated from the social realities and life experiences of millions of women in the world. Camacho, Castro, and Kaufman (2006), in their study of the indigenous women in Latin America, found that the biomedical model of women's reproductive health that discounts social and cultural influences still prevails in the world, especially in developing countries.

I. Development of Gender Equality Approach

The gender equality approach to health and demographic behavior was first pronounced in the 1980s. Three publications sparked off this large interest in population research on the subject of the relationship between gender equality and maternal and infant mortality. One of the publications was on the study of the regional variations in infant and child mortality in North and South India by Dyson and Moore (1983). The southern states of India that were characterized by higher levels of female education and economic independence showed lower infant and child mortality rates compared with the northern states of India where infant and child mortality rates were much higher and the levels of female education and economic independence were lower. Based on the finding, Dyson and Moore argued that gender equality in society is perhaps "the single most important element" in explaining the regional variations in infant and child mortality in India (p. 54).

A second publication came from the work of Karen Oppenheim Mason (1984). In examining the factors that were found to have an effect on infant and child mortality, Mason explained that women's education, domestic autonomy, and gainful employment are among the most important contributing causes of infant and child mortality in certain developing countries. Women with greater autonomy and economic independence are more likely to resist traditional and patriarchal beliefs and practices and have more control over their own well-being and that of their children. Women's education and economic independence, to a large extent, can provide them with the social and economic resources to acquire modern medical services and more hygienic forms of child care (Mason 1984).

The third publication that rejuvenated the academic interest in the subject and added to the understanding of the intrinsic relationship between gender equality and maternal and infant mortality came from John Caldwell's (1986) work on the low mortality rates in some poor countries. Those countries or areas, such as Sri Lanka, Kerala (in India), and Costa Rica, where maternal and infant mortality rates were much lower than those in most of the poor countries during the time when Caldwell conducted the study showed a substantial degree of women's decision-making power, a dedication to education for women and girls, and a history of the egalitarian relationship between women and men. According to Caldwell, the ultimate determinants of infant and maternal mortality decrease are those of maternal resources and in Caldwell's words, female autonomy in comparison to that of males "is perhaps central to exceptional mortality declines especially in poor but open societies." (p. 184).

Scholarly work investigating the impact of gender equality on the demographic phenomena of women's reproductive health and maternal and infant mortality started to grow after the 1994 International Conference on Population and Development (ICPD, known as the Cairo Conference) and the 1995 Fourth World Conference on Women (known as the Beijing Conference). As Nafis Sadik (2000) once reminded us, the term reproductive health was unheard of and gender equality was a matter reserved for visionaries only a couple of decades ago. It is only recently that scholarly investigations about the disparities in health achievement, particularly in women's reproductive health associated with gender equality, have become one of the central themes. Rebecca Cook (1995), Susan McDaniel (1996), Ruth Dixon-Mueller (1998), and Carla Obermeyer (1999) all argued that women's reproductive health cannot be fully achieved without the removal of the socially conditioned barriers and the enhancement of gender equality, especially in less developed and poor countries.

II. Implications of Gender Equality Approach

In sociological terms, gender is a social category marked by unequal access to material and nonmaterial resources between women and men. In this sense, the gender equality approach to women's reproductive health, first of all, requires moving beyond the biomedical model, the conventional sex role theory, and the neo-Malthusian perspective, but focusing on social injustice and structural barriers that directly affect women's reproductive health. As the 2006 World Report on Women's Health (issued by the International Federation of Gynecology and Obstetrics – FIGO) announced, future improvements in women's health, particularly in women's reproductive health, require not only improved medical technology and access to health care, but more importantly, social justice for women and the removal of socially and culturally conditioned barriers to women's equal opportunities. Caldwell (1992) called it an ideological movement in which social scientists, political parties, and medical professionals have important roles to play.

This is not to imply that modern medical technology should be ruled out in explaining maternal and infant health. As Caldwell (1992) noted, the possibility that health transition could have proceeded without technology is slim. Nor is it meant to imply that gender equality will act wholly and alone in retarding maternal and infant mortality and in improving women's reproductive health conditions. The gender equality approach implies that we must go beyond biomedical revelations about women's reproductive functions and, instead look into the social and structural factors that affect women's life experiences and their health conditions as well (Cottingham and Myntti 2002). Cook (1995, 2003) and Cook and Bernard (2003), along with a number of other social scientists, argued that women's reproductive health and their health in general are not just a biological or medical matter nor is it determined by chance genetic inheritance, but most importantly, it is affected by the social and structural environment, namely, social justice for women.

To enhance the gender equality approach to women's reproductive health, therefore, is to acknowledge that reproduction is deeply embedded in the existing social, and including the state, the market, and the family, and that these are the major factors that impinge upon women's opportunities in education, employment, and political participation, and further undermine their reproductive health and the well-being of their children (Morrison and Jutting 2005, Moussa 2008). In a study on gender gap in occupational role attainment, for example, Pratto and Stallworth (1997) and Cotter, Hermsen, Joan, Ovadia, and Vinneman (2001) found that the existing occupational systems and the hiring processes act together to perpetuate a system of gender inequality, where men disproportionately hold "hierarchy-enhancing roles" for their economic, political, and social benefits. In most developing countries, women are still short of access to credit and other economic, social, and political activities necessary for their own well-being and that of their children. Medel-Anonuevo (1995) pointed out that we are still living in the age of "first woman Supreme Court Judge" or "first woman president" of a university. The reproductive role of women in the creation and maintenance of families has been frequently used as grounds to justify the denial of women's equal opportunities. The belief that women are distinguishable from men only with regard to their biological constitution and reproductive roles is still prevalent in many parts of the world, all of which are at the cost of the well-being of women and of their children, particularly women's reproductive health.

In addition, the gender equality approach recognizes that women's reproductive health is directly affected by the value placed on women by the community in which women live. Cook (1995) and Mason (2003) once wrote that women's reproductive health and health in general are heavily influenced by the value system about women and gender relations that is generated by the community. Motherhood and pregnancy can take a woman to the heights of ecstasy and the depths of despair, all depending on the community in which they live as Cook (1995) wrote. Community has been found to be a far stronger mechanism than any individual traits that serves as agents to perpetuate the denial of women's equal opportunities to seek for their own achievements and the satisfaction in the care of their children and their own well-being. Pratto, Stallworth, Sidanius, and Siers (1997) explained that socially and culturally enacted and shared ideas and beliefs about women as well as related ideologies in the community act together to validate a social system of inequalities that is perhaps the largest kind of social injustice against women.

Furthermore, to enhance the gender equality approach to women's reproductive health is to acknowledge that "a gender perspective that more broadly relates gender system to demographic behavior in an international context, and incorporates development issues at large, has emerged only recently" and that "this research is limited in scope and fragmented." (Presser 1997, Hanefeld, Spicer, Brugha, and Walt 2007). Mason and Smith (2003), meanwhile, maintained that the change in approach from a biomedical model to a gender equality approach that emerged during the last decade has just started to turn "what was once viewed as a backwater women's topic … toward the center of demographic enquiry." (p. 3). Sen, George, and Östlin (2002), further pointed out that "Deep-seated gender biases in health research and in policy institutions" in combination with "the lack of well-articulated and accessible evidence" have created a "vicious circle that downgrades the importance of the value of gender perspectives in health." (ix, Preface). It is true that one of the dynamic perceptions of the late 20th century was the growing recognition of the unjust exclusion of women through gender stereotyping and institutional practices, which directly affects women's reproductive health. To a large extent, however, we are still lacking sufficient knowledge about how gender equality or other social inequalities relate to demographic processes, such as pregnancy-related mortality and morbidity and women's reproductive health conditions in particular, in spite of all of the rhetoric that has advocated the empowerment of women and gender equality to advance women's reproductive health. Social scientists and policy makers have acknowledged that this deficiency and lack of knowledge have hindered the progress to improve women's reproductive health and compromised its usefulness to policy makers.

Mann (1996, 1997) and Gostin (2000) have recognized that the gender equality approach will provide a useful framework for understanding and analyzing the social and structural roots of reproductive health and the obligations of the state government to implement social policies for women to obtain equal opportunities for a wide variety of economic, political, and social resources. The study of women's reproductive health and the use of gender equality as an explanatory variable have offered a challenging opportunity for social scientists to make significant contributions to the understanding of the social forces that directly affect women's reproductive health. Sen, George, and Östlin (2002) pointed out in their book titled *Engendering International Health: The Challenge of Equity*, that the gender analysis of health and women's reproductive health in particular that emerged from its infancy in the late 1990s has yet to mature into a perspective that will eventually influence the mainstream thinking in international health and women's reproductive health in particular.

6.2 Engendering Social Policies in Light of Women's Reproductive Health

Social policies are motivated by perceived social problems. A social policy can be understood as a series of public policies designed to achieve a specified set of goals and objectives to promote or impede social change and development. Lister (2000, 2005) pointed out that social policies are mostly defined in terms of un-gendered analysis. As a result, women are more likely to be marginalized than men are. Overwhelming evidence from social science research has shown gender differences in morbidity and mortality and the gap has been the largest in developing countries. According to *The State of World Population* report by the United Nations Fund for Population Activities (UNFPA 2008), health disparity between women and men, particularly in reproductive health related morbidity and mortality, has increased especially in developing countries. Maternal and infant mortality continues to be among the worst performing health indicators in poor countries and regions in spite of the progress that has been achieved since the 1990s (Say, Souza, and Patterson 2009).

Starting in the mid-1990s, the question of how changes in social policies can affect women's health and their reproductive health in particular started to become more pressing (Sen, George, and Östlin 2002) compared with the previous decade when the religious right movement wielded power in the United States and some of the developing countries. The politically mobilized fundamentalist Christian groups saw changes associated with feminism and women's demands for equality and reproductive rights as threatening "the values of the family" and they strongly opposed to women's reproductive rights and reproductive health-related services. At the 1984 World Population Conference, known as the Mexico City Conference, United States President Ronald Reagan announced that the USAID (the United States Agency for International Development) funding would be pulled out from foreign non-governmental organizations (NGOs) that used the funds to address abortion related services and activities, including counseling, referrals, and lobbying to make abortion legal, even though foreign NGOs used their own non-US funds to perform legal abortion services, or provide counseling and referrals, or engage in abortion policy debate. The Mexico City policy (known as the Global Gag Rule) contained three basic restrictions (Cincotta and Crane 2001). First, the policy withheld the USAID family planning grants and technical assistance from foreign NGOs, including reproductive health organizations, women's groups, private hospitals and clinics, and health research centers. Second, the policy imposed a set of restrictions on foreign recipient NGOs, mostly those in developing countries, in terms of family planning and reproductive health services and counseling. And third, the policy prevented foreign recipient NGOs from conducting, with non-US funds, reproductive health related public information campaigns. The Mexico City Policy was later rescinded by US President Clinton in 1993 and the Policy was re-introduced when George W. Bush became President in 2001 (Appendix G. Global Gag Rule Timeline). In 2009, US President Barack Obama issued a memorandum that overturned the Mexico City Policy (Appendix H. President Obama Memorandum to the Secretary of the State and the Administrator of the United States Agency for International Development. January 23, 2009).

The United States has been the single largest donor to international development and by far the largest donor to international family planning programs since the1960s. When we think about the fact that about 200 million women, mostly in developing countries, suffer from pregnancy- and childbirth-related life-threatening complications and disabilities and that pregnancy and childbirth are the leading causes of death and disability for women of reproductive age in developing countries, the impact of the Mexico City Policy is bound to have a tremendous impact on women's reproductive health. John Blane and Matthew Friedman (1990) released a report commissioned by the USAID on the implementation of the Mexico City Policy in Bangladesh, Pakistan, Brazil, Kenya, Turkey, and Egypt. In their 90-page report, they concluded that the fear of losing the USAID funding on the part of most cooperating agencies and foreign non-governmental organizations (NGOs) has led to "overcautiousness" concerning which activities are permitted under the Mexico City Policy and that this caution had caused many foreign NGOs to avoid permitted activities, which "may be having an effect on women's health issues in some cases." (p. 29).

The passage of the Mexico City Policy has translated into the loss of considerable funding for international non-governmental organizations. The International Planned Parenthood Federation (IPPF) reported losing millions of dollars for its member associations, mostly those in developing countries. The Family Planning Association of Kenya, for example, had to close three clinics as a result of the loss of funds from the USAID. Marie Stopes Kenya had to close two clinics after losing an expected $75,000 for its five-year project and the ending of its three-year agreement of 1.6 million dollars with the USAID (Hwang and Stewart 2004). International organizations, such as the World Health Organization (WHO) and the United Nations Fund for Population Activities (UNFPA) were also affected by the policy. As the world's largest internationally funded source of population assistance to developing countries, UNFPA lost 34 million US dollars, amounting to 12 percent of its budget. As a result, UNFPA had to cut back on programs in 20 developing countries, thus leading to the closing of numerous reproductive health centers and clinics, 2 million unwanted pregnancies, and increases in maternal and infant mortality (Alan Guttmacher Institute, Population Reference Bureau, and Population Action International 2003, Hwang and Stewart 2004). Crane and Dusenberry (2004) pointed out that the Mexico City Policy initiated by the United States government in 1984 under Ronald Reagan's presidency and reinforced in 2001 when George W. Bush became the President has interfered with the autonomy and private decision making of the NGOs and violated medical ethics and the human rights of pregnant women. The Policy has directly affected the lives of millions of women and their children, especially those of developing countries and it is even more damaging now than when it was first introduced two decades ago (Crane and Dusenberry 2004, Hwang and Stewart 2004).

The Mexico City Policy serves as an effective example to recognize the responsibilities of the United States government and international non-governmental organizations (NGOs) for implementing international policies in support of a global environment to promote gender equality and women's reproductive health. (Appendix I. List of Selected Non-governmental Organizations: Women's Reproductive Health and Reproductive Rights). As Medel-Anonuevo (1995), Sen, George, and Östlin (2002), and Lister (2005) argued, engendering social policies requires the removal of all social and structural barriers to women's reproductive health, providing everyone with "the enjoyment of the highest attainable standard of the total well-being," (Art. 12, 993 U.N.T.S. 3., 1976) and "the conditions that would ensure all medical services and medical attention in the event of sickness." (Art. 12-2. 1976). The United Nations General Assembly (1999) described the responsibilities of the government and international organizations as taking measures to improve women's social, economic, and political status and "obstetric care, prevention and management of reproductive tract infections, including sexually transmitted diseases" (Paragraph

63). Cook (1995) and Sen, George, and Östlin (2002) further pointed out that a central promise of engendering social policies lies in the government effectively addressing the value of women that extends beyond motherhood and services in the home, removing all the socially constructed barriers, and fulfilling the needs of the poor and the marginalized, most of whom are women. Engendering social policies, therefore, represents a collective and most often, political attempt on the part of the government and international organizations to reconstruct and re-gender those institutions, relations, and discourses in ways that better reflect the perspectives and needs of women (Sen, George, and Östlin 2002).

Lister (2000, 2005) and Sen, George, and Östlin (2002) suggested that engendering social policies in light of women's reproductive health should be understood in the following ways. First, it provides a lens through which to describe and analyze social and population policies along the lines of gender relations. Feminist scholars and social scientists have questioned some of the current social policies in developing countries that have resulted in the vulnerability of women's reproductive health and their well-being. They have pointed out that, regardless of various international efforts, extensive discrimination against women continues to exist. Women's biological constitution and reproductive roles are often being used as justifications for systematic and persistent denial of women's equal opportunities for and their access to social, economic, and political resources. Medicine and medical diagnoses still retain the marks of male dominance under the disguise to protect women. The hierarchical ordering within the social institutions, including the government, the educational system, and organized religion, all reflect the gendered difference of male dominance and female inferiority. In this sense, the government and the state are a gendered institution, reinforcing and regulating unequal gender relations in the interest of men and promoting traditional gender relations through its programs and political agenda, while at the same time generating political clouts to continue for women to be both welfare state workers and users (Fox-Piven 1990, Fox-Harding 1996).

Second, social and economic policies have all too often treated the family as a closed box, into which resources are channeled without any concerns for what happens to the well-being of women and their children. For example, in the field of environmental health, air pollution standards and testing have long ignored the indoor air pollution which is critical for the health of women and their children (Sen, George, and Östlin 2002). In some developing countries, a woman's request for reproductive health care can only be accepted with the authorization of her husband. According to the 2009 State of the Mothers Report, over 70 percent of the 130 million children in the world who are out of school are girls. These girls fail to complete primary school either because they drop out in early grades or because they never get the chance to attend school (Save the Children 2009).

Third, social policies need to take seriously the issues of women's economic dependence on men and their social and political status in society. Ferree (1990), in an analysis of gender and the family, pointed out that families continue to operate in ways to maintain women's subordination through processes of women's economic dependence on men. Although women spend about 70 percent of their unpaid time caring for family members, this contribution to the global economy remains invisible (United Nations Development Programme 2006). Of the world's 1 billion poorest people, three-fifths are women and girls. Everywhere, women typically earn less than men, both because they are concentrated in low-paying jobs and because they are paid less for the same work. Of the 960 million adults in the world who cannot read or write, two-thirds are women. Women are conspicuously absent from parliaments, making up on average only 16 percent of parliamentarians worldwide (United Nations Development Programme 2006). Wilkinson (1996), Macintyre (1997), and Breen (2002) argued that engendering social policies in light of women's reproductive health implies that social policies should be assessed with regards to their effect on women's social, economic, and political gains and the well-being of their children. Unfortunately, some development policies, such as economic adjustment policies and development programs especially those in developing and poor countries often failed to recognize women's economic conditions and their capacities as agents for change and equitable health outcomes (Bangser 2002).

Recently, Breen (2002) and Sen and the colleagues (2002), suggested "gender planning" as a social policy component for developing practical strategies to promote gender equality and address the advancement of women's health and reproductive health in particular. That is, not only should the social policy at issue be guaranteed in laws and practices, but there should be mechanisms and procedures in place for women to defend themselves in the event of violations.

In population studies, academic endeavors and actual social policies are, to a large extent, more inextricably tied together than any other aspects of social sciences. According to Basu (2000), Mason and Smith (2003), and World Health Organization (WHO 2008), demographic research on the social determinants of fertility, mortality, and health remains inseparable from the development of theoretical explanations and the formation of effective social policies to address the health condition of a population and, in particular, women's reproductive health. Over the decades, some progress has been made due to international effort and demographic studies on fertility, mortality, and health transition, both of which have contributed to the changing world view of the social and economic roots of women's reproductive health. As Sadik (2000) argued, today there is some general agreement that population processes of fertility and mortality are a key development issue, inextricably linked with economic progress, social justice, and gender equality. Reproductive health and gender equality are becoming part of the international agenda as specified in the Millennium Development Goals (MDGs). In spite of the progress, however, there is still a long way to go to implement social policies that would enhance gender equality and further improve women's reproductive health. Some feminist scholars and activists still remain skeptical about the existing masculinized and hierarchical social systems given the fact that gender inequality and social injustice are heavily embedded within the current social, political and economic systems.

Actions to implement social policies involve shared global alliances and partnerships, including all countries and health organizations to generate adequate investment and effective strategies. According to the United Nations (2009), in 2008, about 0.30 percent of developed countries' combined national income was contributed to OECD's (Organization for Economic Co-opearation and Development) official development assistance (ODA) fund (Appendix J. Countries in Major World Aggregates). The United States was the largest donor by amount in 2008, followed by Germany, the United Kingdom, France, and Japan (United Nations 2009). However, the total percentage of the aid to the poorest developing countries remains well below the United Nations target of 0.7 percent of gross national income[1] (Appendix K. Countries or Areas in Income Aggregates). The only countries that reached or exceeded the United Nations target in 2008 were Denmark, Luxemburg, the Netherlands, Norway, and Sweden.

Health is knowledge based and socially driven (Chen et al. 2004). The knowledge is not just that of new medicine and medical technologies, but also that about people. As Basu (2000) and Lewis (2000) proposed, engendering social policies, on the one hand, involves creating an agenda to empower women and ensure gender equality across numerous social divisions and national boundaries; and on the other hand, it requires that social policies recognize the specificity of particular relations of inequality and be assessed with regard to their effect on women's social, economic, and political gains that directly affect women's reproductive health and their well-being.

6.3 Limitations of the Study

This study has certain limitations that need to be addressed.

I. Selection of Indicators

Presser (1997) maintained that a deeper understanding of the complex relationships between women's reproductive health and explanatory variables requires both the availability and the quality of quantitative data bases and innovative methodologies. The greater the data availability on women's reproductive health and relevant variables, the more feasible it is to assess reproductive health programs and to improve women's reproductive health at large.

Data availability, however, has been inadequate, especially for developing countries. Sims and Butter (2000, 2002) claimed that the absence of systematic and rigorous data is most stark in poor countries and for poor women. This is partly due to problems related to the sources of information (Zuray, Khattab, Younis, El-Mouelhy, and Fadle 1993). First, statistics from health institutions in developing countries generally suffer from problems of incomplete coverage.

1 The poorest countries are those countries classified as "least developed countries" (LDCs) or low or low-middle income countries. The 49 least developed countries receive about one third of all aid fund (United Nations 2009).

This problem is particularly severe when women's health is concerned simply because of the lack of support for women to visit health services and the culture of silence among women regarding their health especially their reproductive health (Dixon-Mueller and Wasserheit 1991, Khattab 1992, Zuray, Khattab, Younis, El-Mouelhy, and Fadle 1993). In addition, most population-based surveys directed at women in developing countries have largely concentrated on issues other than women's health and reproductive health, such as maternal and child health (Zuray, Khattab, Younis, El-Mouelhy, and Fadle 1993, United Nations Fund for Population Activities – UNFPA 2003).

As data of more relevant indicators become available and validated by the accumulation of empirical findings, the number of scale items may be expanded and the value of alpha is likely to increase.

II. Conceptualizing Variables in Multinational Research

In spite of the ever-increasing responsiveness to the issue of gender equality, women's rights, and reproductive health, rendering definitions of these concepts that are meaningful across populations has been highly controversial in international conferences and conventions and among academic researchers. Penna and Campbell (1998), for example, questioned the universality of the human rights concept and suggested that the Western concept of human rights may not be applicable to non-Western cultures and societies, especially when dealing with the rights of women. In discussing the cultural context of reproductive health, Obermeyer (1999) argued for a cultural perspective that incorporates "the concerns of very different constituencies," that is, those "who formulate and implement policies" and "those who are the targets of policies." (p. 50).

Clark (1991) and Blanc (2001), however, challenged those who see gender-based power relations as a component of culture which is perceived as nebulous, static, untouchable, and impermeable to interventions and changes. Gupta (2000) wrote that many scholars and policy makers are hesitant to intervene in academic discussions of gender-related norms for fear of being labeled culturally insensitive and disrespectful of tradition.

Given the different approaches to conceptualizing variables, such as gender equality, women's rights, and reproductive health in cross-country research, social scientists will face substantial challenges in future research. According to Hansluwka (1985) and Zuray and the colleagues (1993), there are four types of difficulties in conceptualizing variables in multinational research: vagueness of the concept, value judgment of the definer, multidimensionality of the phenomenon, and the impossibility of meaningful operationalization.

For this study, the conceptual framework and the selection of the scale items used to measure all of the variables in this study were determined after an extensive review of the related literature. For future research, the meaning of a particular concept or behavior within or across a particular social and cultural context is likely to change over time. As a result, the relevance of a specific concept and indicator(s) may vary over time and therefore the number of scale items may be deleted or expanded for addition.

III. Impact of Culture

Future research may consider the impact of culture on women's reproductive health. In terms of the conceptualization and the measurement of culture, one can easily find a dearth of clear concepts and measures of the word "culture." Straub, Loch, Evaristo, Karahanna, and Srite (2002) called culture a "thorny concept and even thornier research conduct." (p. 14). It is more so to develop measures of culture at an aggregate level. Straub and the colleagues group definitions of culture into three main categories, (1) definitions based on shared values, (2) definitions based on problem solving, and (3) general all-encompassing definitions.

Given the complexity in defining culture and the operational tools by which culture is measured as a scientific construct, empirical research faces substantial challenges.

IV. Cross Sectional Data

Studies on women's reproductive health have employed a variety of methods, such as surveys, interviews, and clinical examinations, which have elicited empirical, descriptive, and clinical results. The majority of the studies are cross-sectional in nature. The cross-sectional nature of the research may impose some uncertainty in terms of a clear-cut causal attribution. Although a clear-cut causal attribution might be shaky if one uses cross-sectional data, still, as Jameson (1996) and Pearl (2000) admitted, generating cause-effect relationships among variables is the fundamental building block of empirical research and empirical research using cross-sectional data can make substantial contributions to the understanding of social issues and to social policy resolutions.

6.4 Summary

Presser (1997), Blanc (2001), and Östlin (2004) pointed out that one of the deficiencies of research to date is the small number of rigorous quantitative models that specify the link between gender-based power relations and sexual and reproductive health outcomes in an international context and incorporate development issues at large. This book features an empirical study and presents discussions on the conceptualization and the operational indicators of all of the variables used in this study (Chapter 3 Measurement of the Variables). In addition, this book explores the effects of gender equality, women's human rights, and maternal-child care on women's reproductive health in the context of economic and political development. Inferences are drawn from data obtained from 137 developing countries (or areas). Structural equation analysis is used to test the proposed model.

Empirical findings from the proposed model indicate the importance of gender equality and maternal-child care in predicting women's reproductive health in developing countries. The effect of gender equality and maternal-child care on women's reproductive health is strong and statistically significant ($p<.01$). The empirical findings have provided certain useful insight that women's reproductive health is inextricably linked to gender equality. This finding is consistent with the thesis that the achievement of women's reproductive health depends on a social environment where women are provided with equal access to social, economic, and political resources. To better understand the impact of gender equality on women's reproductive health, first, it is important to recognize that inequalities in society raise mortality by restricting or reducing access of the powerless to social resources, including political decision making, education, occupational prestige, and financial gains. Second, in more egalitarian societies, women have more control over their own social, economic, and political resources, which is essential for creating an environment where women can achieve their reproductive goals and improve their reproductive health conditions.

The finding that there is a significant and direct relationship between maternal-child care and women's reproductive health may permit a possible verification for effective maternal and child care given the current social conditions in developing countries, particularly the neglect of the health needs of many of the women and their children.

The women's human rights hypothesis is not supported by the data from the 137 developing countries. In this study, women's human rights are measured by two variables, legal status of abortion right and women's political, economic, and social rights (Chapter 3 Measurement of the Variables). It is perhaps that human rights provide a legal discourse for political functions and social welfare issues but that the legally binding human rights instruments may not be sufficient to provide a moral and social foundation for the attainment of human well-being and women's reproductive health. A formal legal approach may not be adequate to lead to women's reproductive health as measured in this study. This finding casts certain doubts about the claims pronounced at recent international conferences and conventions.

Economic development is found to be positively related to gender equality and maternal-child care. This finding suggests a more or less linear improvement in gender equality in developing countries as a result of economic development. It is perhaps that economic growth, as a form of technological advancement and liberal ideology, can serve to redress gender equality in developing countries as a whole.

In addition, the findings from the multiple regression analysis indicate that sub-Saharan African countries as a whole are facing major challenges to reduce pregnancy-related deaths and to improve women's reproductive health in comparison with the other regions under study (Arab states, East Asia/Pacific, South Asia, and Latin American/Caribbean). The challenges to improve the reproductive health of millions of African women are more daunting than those in the other regions included in this study. The case of sub-Saharan Africa serves as ample evidence of widening health inequalities across the region and between regions of developing countries

On May 22, 2009, the World Health Assembly passed a resolution on "reducing health inequalities through action on social determinants of health" and pushed for new research priorities to address the social determinants of health, including social hierarchies and gender equality, and broader social, political, and economic factors (Östlin, Schrecker, and Sadana 2009). The findings from the 137 developing countries in this study are in line with the resolution of the World Health Assembly. The gender equality approach, in contrast to biomedical and neo-Malthusian perspectives, lies at the core of social justice for women (Rose 1994, Camacho, Castro, and Kaufman 2006, Keleher and Franklin 2008). It seeks to reconstruct the main variables that directly affect women's health in general and reproductive health in particular. It, therefore, provides a new and useful framework in the analysis of women's reproductive health. It is highly likely that the women-centered gender equality approach that incorporates economic development measures in an international context of developing countries will spur on more scholarly endeavor to redress inadequacies in research on the social determinants of women's reproductive health and will, at the same time, create more challenging opportunities for the international community to confront the unprecedented crises in women's reproductive health in the poor countries of the world.

Appendix A

Millennium Development Goals (MDGs), Targets, and Indicators[1]

Goal 1. Eradicate extreme poverty and hunger

Target 1.A: Reduce half, between 1990 and 2015, the proportion of people whose income is less than one dollar a day

- 1.1 Proportion of population below $1 (PPP) per day
- 1.2 Poverty gap ratio
- 1.3 Share of poorest quintile in national consumption

Target 1.B: Achieve full and productive employment and decent work for all, including women and young people

- 1.4 Growth rate of GDP per person employed
- 1.5 Employment-to-population ratio
- 1.6 Proportion of employed people living below $1 (PPP) per day
- 1.7 Proportion of own-account and contributing family workers in total employment

Target 1.C: Reduce half, between 1990 and 2015, the proportion of people who suffer from hunger

- 1.8 Prevalence of underweight children under-five years of age
- 1.9 Proportion of population below minimum level of dietary energy consumption

Goal 2: Achieve universal primary education

Target 2.A: Ensure that, by 2015, children everywhere, boys and girls alike, will be able to complete a full course of primary schooling

- 2.1 Net enrolment ratio in primary education
- 2.2 Proportion of pupils starting grade 1 who reach last grade of primary education
- 2.3 Literacy rate of 15–24 year-olds, women and men

1 Effective 15 January 2008.

Goal 3: Promote gender equality and empower women

Target 3.A: Eliminate gender disparity in primary and secondary education, preferably by 2005, and in all levels of education no later than 2015

- 3.1 Ratios of girls to boys in primary, secondary, and tertiary education
- 3.2 Share of women in wage employment in the non-agricultural sector
- 3.3 Proportion of seats held by women in national parliament

Goal 4: Reduce child mortality

Target 4.A: Reduce by two-thirds, between 1990 and 2015, the under-five mortality rate

- 4.1 Under-five mortality rate
- 4.2 Infant mortality rate
- 4.3 Proportion of one-year-old children immunized against measles

Goal 5: Improve maternal health

Target 5.A: Reduce by three quarters, between 1990 and 2015, the maternal mortality ratio

- 5.1 Maternal mortality ratio
- 5.2 Proportion of births attended by skilled health personnel

Target 5.B: Achieve, by 2015, universal access to reproductive health

- 5.3 Contraceptive prevalence rate
- 5.4 Adolescent birth rate
- 5.5 Antenatal care coverage (at least one visit and at least four visits)
- 5.6 Unmet need for family planning

Goal 6: Combat HIV/AIDS, malaria, and other diseases

Target 6.A: Have halted by 2015 and begun to reverse the spread of HIV/AIDS

- 6.1 HIV prevalence among population aged 15–24 years
- 6.2 Condom use at last high-risk sex
- 6.3 Proportion of population aged 15–24 years with comprehensive correct knowledge of HIV/AIDS
- 6.4 Ratio of school attendance of orphans to school attendance of non-orphans aged 10–14 years

Target 6.B: Achieve, by 2010, universal access to treatment for HIV/AIDS for all those who need it

6.5 Proportion of population with advanced HIV infection with access to anti-retroviral drugs

Target 6.C: Have halted, by 2015, and begun to reverse the incidence of malaria and other major diseases

6.6 Incidence and death rates associated with malaria
6.7 Proportion of children under five sleeping under insecticide-treated bednets
6.8 Proportion of children under five with fever who are treated with appropriate anti-malarial drugs
6.9 Incidence, prevalence, and death rates associated with tuberculosis
6.10 Proportion of tuberculosis cases detected and cured under directly observed treatment short course

Goal 7: Ensure environmental sustainability

Target 7.A: Integrate the principles of sustainable development into country policies and programmes and reverse the loss of environmental resources

Target 7.B: Reduce biodiversity loss, achieving, by 2010, a significant reduction in the rate of loss

7.1 Proportion of land area covered by forest
7.2 CO2 emissions, total, per capita and per $1 GDP (PPP)
7.3 Consumption of ozone-depleting substances
7.4 Proportion of fish stocks within safe biological limits
7.5 Proportion of total water resources used
7.6 Proportion of terrestrial and marine areas protected
7.7 Proportion of species threatened with extinction

Target 7.C: Reduce by half, by 2015, the proportion of people without sustainable access to safe drinking water and basic sanitation

7.8 Proportion of population using an improved drinking water source
7.9 Proportion of population using an improved sanitation facility

Target 7.D: By 2020, to have achieved a significant improvement in the lives of at least 100 million slum dwellers

7.10 Proportion of urban population living in slums

Goal 8: Develop a global partnership for development

Target 8.A: Develop further an open, rule-based, predictable, non-discriminatory trading and financial system

Includes a commitment to good governance, development, and poverty reduction – both nationally and internationally

Target 8.B: Address the special needs of the least developed countries

Includes: tariff and quota free access for the least developed countries' exports; enhanced programme of debt relief for heavily indebted poor countries (HIPC) and cancellation of official bilateral debt; and more generous ODA for countries committed to poverty reduction.

Target 8.C: Address the special needs of landlocked developing countries and small island developing States (through the Programme of Action for the Sustainable Development of Small Island Developing States and the outcome of the twenty-second special session of the General Assembly)

Target 8.D: Deal comprehensively with the debt problems of developing countries through national and international measures in order to make debt sustainable in the long term

Some of the indicators listed below are monitored separately for the least developed countries (LDCs), Africa, landlocked developing countries and small island developing States.

Official development assistance (ODA)

8.1 Net ODA, total and to the least developed countries, as percentage of OECD/DAC donors' gross national income
8.2 Proportion of total bilateral, sector-allocable ODA of OECD/DAC donors to basic social services (basic education, primary health care, nutrition, safe water, and sanitation)
8.3 Proportion of bilateral official development assistance of OECD/DAC donors that is untied
8.4 ODA received in landlocked developing countries as a proportion of their gross national incomes
8.5 ODA received in small island developing States as a proportion of their gross national incomes

Market access

8.6 Proportion of total developed country imports (by value and excluding arms) from developing countries and least developed countries, admitted free of duty
8.7 Average tariffs imposed by developed countries on agricultural products and textiles and clothing from developing countries
8.8 Agricultural support estimate for OECD countries as a percentage of their gross domestic product
8.9 Proportion of ODA provided to help build trade capacity

Debt sustainability

8.10 Total number of countries that have reached their HIPC decision points and number that have reached their HIPC completion points (cumulative)

8.11 Debt relief committed under HIPC and MDRI Initiatives

8.12 Debt service as a percentage of exports of goods and services

Target 8.E: In cooperation with pharmaceutical companies, provide access to affordable essential drugs in developing countries

8.13 Proportion of population with access to affordable essential drugs on a sustainable basis

Target 8.F: In cooperation with the private sector, make available the benefits of new technologies, especially information and communications

8.14 Telephone lines per 100 population

8.15 Cellular subscribers per 100 population

8.16 Internet users per 100 population

The Millennium Development Goals and targets came from the Millennium Declaration, signed by 189 countries, including 147 heads of State and Government, in September 2000 (http://www.un.org/millennium/declaration/ares552e.htm) and from further agreement by member states at the 2005 World Summit (Resolution adopted by the General Assembly – A/RES/60/1, http://www.un.org/Docs/journal/asp/ws.asp?m=A/RES/60/1).

* Effective of January 2008, MDG monitoring framework was revised to include four new targets: Target 1.B, Target 5.B, Target 6.B, and Target 7.B.

Sources

World Bank. 2008. *Official List of MDG Indicators*. Available at: http://siteresources.worldbank.org/datastatistics/resources/MDGsOfficialList2008.pdf.

United Nations (UN). 2009. *The Millennium Development Goals Report 2009*. Available at: www.un.org/millenniumgoals/pdf/MDG_Report_2009_EN.pdf.

Appendix B
Declaration of the Rights of Man and the Citizen, 26 August 1789

The representatives of the French people, constituted as a National Assembly, and considering that ignorance, neglect, or contempt of the rights of man are the sole causes of public misfortunes and government corruption, have resolved to set forth in a solemn declaration of the natural, inalienable and sacred rights of man: so that by being constantly present to all the members of the social body this declaration may always remind them of their rights and duties; so that by being liable at every moment to comparison with the aim of any and all political institutions the acts of the legislative and executive powers may be the more fully respected: and so that by being founded henceforward on simple and incontestable principles the demands of the citizens may always tend toward maintaining the constitution and the general welfare.

In consequence, the National Assembly recognizes and declares: in the presence and under the auspices of the Supreme Being, the following rights of man and the citizen:

1. Men are born and remain free and equal in rights. Social distinctions may be based only on common utility.
2. The purpose of all political association is the preservation of the natural and imprescriptible rights of man. These rights are liberty, property, security, and resistance to oppression.
3. The principle of all sovereignty rests essentially in the nation. Nobody and no individual may exercise authority which does not emanate expressly from the nation.
4. Liberty consists in the ability to do whatever does not harm another; hence the exercise of the natural rights of each man has no other limits than those which assure to other members of society the employment of the same rights. These limits can only be determined by the law.
5. The law only has the right to prohibit those actions which are injurious to society. No hindrance should be put in the way of anything not prohibited by the law, nor may any one be forced to do what the law does not require.
6. The law is the expression of the general will. All citizens have the right to take part, in person or by their representatives, in its formation. It must be the same for everyone whether it protects or penalizes. All citizens being equal in its eyes are equally admissible to all public dignities, offices, and

employments, according to their ability, and with no other distinction than that of their virtues and talents.

7. No man may be indicted, arrested, detained except in cases determined by the law and according to the forms which it has prescribed. Those who seek, expedite, execute, or cause to be executed arbitrary orders should be punished; but citizens summoned or seized by virtue of the law should obey instantly, and render themselves guilty by resistance.
8. Only strictly and obviously necessary punishments may be established by the law, and no one may be punished except by virtue of a law established and promulgated before the time of the offense, and legally applied.
9. Every man being presumed innocent until judged guilty, if it is deemed indispensable to arrest him, all rigor unnecessary to securing his person should be severely repressed by law.
10. No one should be disturbed for his opinions, even in religion, provided that their manifestation does not trouble public order as established by law.
11. The free communication of thoughts and opinions is one of the most precious of the rights of man. Every citizen may therefore speak, write, and print freely, if he accepts his own responsibility for any abuse of this liberty in the cases set by the law.
12. The safeguard of the rights of man and the citizen requires public powers. These powers are therefore instituted for the advantage of all, and not for the private benefit of those to whom they are entrusted.
13. For maintenance of public authority and for expenses of administration, common taxation is indispensable. It should be apportioned equally among all citizens according to their capacity to pay.
14. All citizens have the right, by themselves or through their representatives, to have demonstrated to them the necessity of public taxes, to consent to them freely, to follow the use made of the proceeds, and to determine the means of apportionment, assessment, and collection, and the duration of them.
15. Society has the right to hold accountable every public agent of the administration.
16. Any society in which the guarantee of rights is not assured or the separation of powers not settled has no constitution.
17. Property being an inviolable and sacred right, no one may be deprived of it except when public necessity, certified by law, obviously requires it, and on the condition of a just compensation in advance.

Source

The French Revolution and Human Rights: A Brief Documentary History (translated, edited, and with an Introduction by Lynn Hunt).1996: 77–9. Boston/New York: Bedford/St. Martin's.

Appendix C

Chronology of International Conferences on Gender Equality, Women's Rights, and Women's Reproductive Health

1948: United Nations approved the Universal Declaration of Human Rights
The Declaration spelled out for the first time a global agreement that every woman, man, and child has certain rights merely because they are human beings. No exceptions for cultural norms, national traditions, family matters, or religious teachings. No exceptions for gender, skin color, ethnicity, religious or political views, or nationality.

1968: First International Conference on Human Rights, Tehran
The conference recognized that "Parents have a basic human right to decide freely and responsibly the number and spacing of their children and a right to adequate education and information to do so."

1969: The United Nations Fund for Population Activities (UNFPA) was created.

1974: First World Population Conference, Bucharest
The conference launched the first World Population Year and put population issues on the international agenda.

1975: First World Conference on Women, Mexico City
The conference declared that the right to family planning is essential for equality between men and women and called for a women's convention to promote equal rights for women worldwide.

The conference set the goals: full gender equality and elimination of gender discrimination, integration and full participation of women in development, and greater involvement of women in strengthening world peace.

1976: The United Nations Development Fund for Women (UNIFEM) was created.

1976–85: UN International Decade for Women
Two thirds of UN member states have since adopted some sort of national "plan" for women.

1979: The United Nations adopted the Convention on the Elimination of all Forms of Discrimination against Women (CEDAW). CEDAW committed signing countries and states to "take all appropriate measures to eliminate discrimination against women" in every area of life, including a guarantee to women of the "right to decide freely and responsibly on the number and spacing of their children and to have access to the information, education, and means to enable them to exercise these rights."

1980: Second World Conference on Women, Copenhagen
The conference listed three priorities: (1) equal access to education, (2) to employment opportunities, and (3) to adequate health care.

1984: International Conference on Population, Mexico City
The conference added individuals to the Teheran description of family planning rights, asserting that unmarried individuals also have the rights to reproductive health services. The conference documented dangers of unsafe abortion and recognized a global unmet need for contraceptive services. In the United States, the Reagan administration announced a "global gag rule" barring US funding for non-US groups advocating or counseling on legal abortion. Other countries joined the debate on abortion access.

1987: Safe Motherhood Conference, Nairobi
The enormous toll of women dying in pregnancy and childbirth worldwide – more than one per minute – led the World Health Organization, the World Bank and United Nations Fund for Population Activities, and the UN Population Fund to spearhead research and advocacy in the Safe Motherhood Initiative to promote investment in saving women's lives. For 20 years, it has contributed to the reduction of maternal mortality, a major health goal for governments worldwide.

1989: The United Nations approved Convention on the Rights of the Child
The convention recognized "... the right of the child to the enjoyment of the highest attainable standard of health and to facilities for the treatment of illness and rehabilitation of health," and committed signing states to developing "... preventive health care, guidance for parents, and family planning education and services."

1992: The United Nations Conference on Environment and Development, Rio de Janeiro The Earth Summit recognized women's vital role in sustainable development and environmental management.

1993: World Conference on Human Rights, Vienna
The conference declared that women's rights are human rights, condemned violence against women as a human rights abuse, and affirmed "a woman's right

to the widest range of family planning services." The conference led to the naming of a special UN rapporteur to monitor abuses of women's rights worldwide. It also recognized "the importance of the enjoyment by women of the highest standard of physical and mental health throughout their life span" (Article 41).

1993: Population Summit of the World's Scientific Academies, New Delhi
The Summit explored in detail the interrelated issues of population growth, resource consumption, socio-economic development, and environmental protection. A statement signed by 58 academies declared that success in dealing with social, economic, and environmental problems depends on achieving a stable world population.

1994, Sept. 5–13: International Conference on Population and Development (ICPD), Cairo
The conference rejected demographic targets in favor of action to meet the needs of individuals for universal education and sexual and reproductive health care and rights as the best road to sustainable development. Leaders of 179 countries agreed on a 20-year Programme of Action – "the Cairo Consensus" – that called for investments in women of $21.7 billion per year by 2015. An NGO Forum aired grassroots groups' ideas on the same issues.

1995: Fourth World Conference on Women, Beijing
The Declaration and the Platform for Action placed women at the center of any successful policy for economic and social development. The documents affirmed adolescents' rights and listed 12 critical areas of concern for achieving equality, development, and peace, setting targets and steps to meet the goals. The UN General Assembly later endorsed both documents.

1995: World Summit on Social Development, Copenhagen
The Summit committed participating countries to work towards providing official development assistance equal to 0.7 percent of gross national income.

1998: Vienna + 5, Rome
The Rome Statute of the International Criminal Court recognized that rape and sexual violence are among the most serious of war crimes.

1999: ICPD + 5, The Hague
As an official UN meeting, it assessed global progress on the ICPD Programme of Action and reaffirmed the Cairo Consensus. The meeting issued recommendations to help meet the 2015 deadline. It found new efforts worldwide to improve women's rights, education, and health care, with family planning use and services up. But funding lags and HIV/AIDS have become a global pandemic. A UN General Assembly Special Session called upon all countries to fulfill their commitments to specific investments in those areas.

2000: Beijing + 5, New York
It reaffirmed principles of both the Cairo Programme of Action and the Beijing Platform for Action. It called for more male involvement in promoting women's rights and sexual and reproductive health and re-stated the importance of integrating a gender perspective into the HIV/AIDS response.

2000: Millennium Development Summit, Declaration, and Millennium Development Goals (MDGs)
World leaders agreed on eight MDGs that focus on halving global poverty by 2015 and summed up the objectives of recent UN conferences, including gender equality and women's empowerment. Each MDG goal set specific targets, such as a three-quarters reduction in maternal deaths and a two-thirds reduction in child deaths.

2001: UN General Assembly Special Session (UNGASS) on HIV/AIDS, New York
A Declaration of Commitment, by far the most comprehensive effort to address the HIV/AIDS pandemic, set many policy recommendations on gender and women's vulnerability. It stressed the urgent need of adolescents worldwide, especially girls and women, for sexual and reproductive health education and services.

2002: World Children's Summit, New York
It called for essential and emergency obstetric care before, during, and after pregnancy and delivery as the best way to save the lives of women and children worldwide.

2002: World Summit on Sustainable Development, Johannesburg
It focused on economic and financial approaches to development rather than on population and rights-based policies.

2004: ICPD + 10
At several meetings, the international community discussed backlash but reaffirmed the ICPD Programme of Action, including many countries that objected to sexual and reproductive rights in 1994. The NGO Countdown 2015 International Roundtable drew more than 700 participants to London to assess progress and express disappointment at the slow pace of policy change and investment in women.

2005: Beijing +10
The UN Commission on the Status of Women found that the Platform for Action had sparked major improvements for women in some places although reaction had worsened conditions in others. Promises of funding and policy change were not being kept. The regional Mexico City Consensus meeting urged governments to implement legislation "guaranteeing the responsible exercise of sexual and

reproductive rights and non-discriminatory access to health services, including sexual and reproductive health…"

2006: The United Nations General Assembly, New York
At the recommendation of the Secretary-General, another target for MDG 5 was noted: improve maternal health: achieve universal access to reproductive health by 2015. It proposed new indicators for measuring progress: adolescent birth rate, antenatal care coverage, unmet need for family planning, and contraceptive prevalence rate. These were adopted in 2007.

2006: African Union Meeting, Mozambique
African Union leaders agreed on the Maputo Plan of Action, which committed them to moving toward universal access to comprehensive sexual and reproductive health services across the continent by 2015.

2007: Women Deliver Conference, London
Nearly 2,000 parliamentarians, activists and women's advocates from 107 countries met to reinvigorate global political will to invest in women as the best way to improve maternal health, reduce child mortality and promote economic development.

2009: ICPD@15
Oct. 12: United Nations General Assembly Special Session to commemorate ICPD @ 15 Oct. 26–27, Addis Ababa: 4th International Parliamentarians' Conference on ICPD implementation.

2010: United Nations, New York: MDG +10 Summit on global progress toward implementing the Millennium Development Goals.

2015: Deadline to attain the ICPD Programme of Action goals and the Millennium Development Goals.

Source

United Nations. 2009. Available at: www.icpdat15.org/assets/pdf/chronology.pdf.

Appendix D
Women's Human Rights and Reproductive Rights

The twelve human rights that are stated in international human rights instruments provide the basis for women's reproductive rights. The first is the right to life (Article 3, Universal Declaration of Human Rights 1948). The International Planned Parenthood Federation (IPPF) (2000) further specified the right to life as the following.

1. No women's life should be put at risk or endangered by reason of pregnancy.
2. No child's life should be put or risk or endangered, particularly not by reason of her/his gender.
3. No person's life should be put at risk or endangered by reason of lack of access to health care services and/or information, counseling or services to sexual or reproductive health.
4. The right of all girl infants to be free from the risk of female infanticide (p. 12).

The second is the right to liberty and security of the person (Article 3, Universal Declaration of Human Rights 1948). The right is indicated by:

1. All persons have the right to be free to enjoy and control their sexual and reproductive life, having due regard to the rights of others.
2. All persons have the right to be free from any medical intervention related to their sexual and reproductive health with their full, free and informed consent.
3. All females have the right to be free from all forms of genital mutilation.
4. All persons have the right to be free from sexual harassment.
5. All persons have the right to be free from externally imposed fear, shame, guilt, beliefs based on myths, and other psychological factors inhibiting their sexual response or impairing their sexual relationships.
6. All persons have the right to be free from forced pregnancy, sterilization and abortion.

(IPPF 2000, 13)

The third right is the right to equality, dignity, and to be free from all forms of discrimination as stated in articles 1 and 7 of the Universal Declaration of Human

Rights (1948). IPPF (2000) recognizes the following rights with regard to women's reproductive rights.

1. No persons should be discriminated against in their sexual and reproductive lives, in their access to health care and/or services on the grounds of race, color, sex or sexual orientation, marital status, family position, age, language, religion, political or other opinion, national or social origin, property, birth or other status.
2. All persons have the right to equal access to education and information to ensure their health and well-being, including access to information, advice and services relating to their sexual and reproductive health and rights, irrespective of race, color, poverty, sex, sexual orientation, marital status, family position, age, language, religion, political or other opinion, national or social origin, poverty, birth or other status.
3. All women and girl children have the right to appropriate nutrition and care throughout their life-span, and to be free prejudicial, customary and all other practices which are based on the idea of inferiority or stereotyped roles for men and women and/or amount to discrimination against them.
4. No woman should be discriminated against in her access to education, information and/or services related either to development, or to her sexual and reproductive health and rights, including access to fertility regulation services, by reason that the consent of another is required.
5. No person should be subjected to any sexual or reproductive health care programme which has the effect of discriminating against particular population groups.
6. All persons have the right to protection from all forms of violence caused by reason of their race, color, sex, language, religion, political or other opinion, national or social origin, property, birth or other status.
7. All women have the right to protection from discrimination in social, domestic or employment spheres by reason of pregnancy or motherhood.
8. No person shall be discriminated against in their access to information, health care, or services related to their sexual and reproductive health, rights and needs, throughout their life-span, on the grounds of gender, age, sexual orientation or mental or physical disability. (pp. 14–15)

The fourth is the right to privacy (Article 12, Universal Declaration of Human Rights, 1948). The attainment of women's reproductive rights with regard to the right to privacy can be realized by ensuring the following rights (IPPF 2000, 16).

1. All sexual and reproductive health care services, including information and counseling, should provide clients with privacy and ensure that personal information given will remain confidential.
2. All women have the right to autonomous reproductive choices including choices relating to safe abortion.

3. All persons have the right to express their sexual orientation in order to have a safe and satisfying sex life, having due regard to well-being and rights of others, without fear of persecution, or denial of liberty or social interference.
4. All sexual and reproductive health care services, including information and counseling services, provided should be made available to all individuals and couples, especially young people, on a basis which respects their rights to privacy and confidentiality.

The fifth is the right to freedom of thought as stated in article 18 of the Universal Declaration of Human Rights (1948). The right is indicated by the following rights with regard to women's reproductive rights (IPPF 2000, 17).

1. All persons have the right to freedom of thought and speech related to their sexual and reproductive lives.
2. All persons have the right to protection against restrictions on grounds of thought, conscience and religion to their access to education and information related to their sexual and reproductive health.
3. Health care professionals have the right to conscientious objection with regard to providing contraception and abortion services only if they can refer the client to health professionals willing to provide the service immediately. No such right exists in emergency cases where lives are at risk.
4. All persons have the right to be free from restrictive interpretation of religious texts, beliefs, philosophies and customs as tools to curtail freedom of thought on sexual and reproductive health care and other issues.

The sixth right is the right to freedom and education (Articles 26, Universal Declaration of Human Rights 1948). IPPF (2000) recognized the following rights as being related to the right to freedom and education.

1. All persons have the right of access to education and correct information related to their sexual and reproductive health, rights and responsibilities which is gender sensitive, free from stereotypes, and presented in an objective, critical and pluralistic manner.
2. All persons have the right to sufficient education and information to ensure that any decisions they make related to their sexual and reproductive life are made with full, free and informed consent.
3. All persons have the right to full information as to the relative benefits, risks and effectiveness of all methods of fertility regulation and the prevention of unplanned pregnancies. (p. 18)

The seventh right is the right to choose whether or not to marry and to found and plan a family (Article 16, Universal Declaration of Human Rights 1948). IPPF (2000) further specifies the right as the following.

1. All persons have the right to protection against a requirement to marry without that person's full, free and informed consent.
2. All persons have the right of access to reproductive health care services including those who are infertile, or whose fertility is jeopardized by sexually transmitted diseases. (p.19)

The eighth right is the right to decide whether or when to have children as stated in article 16, Universal Declaration of Human Rights (1948). The right is indicated by the following rights as specified by IPPF (2000, 20).

1. All women have the right to information, education and services necessary for the protection of reproductive health, safe motherhood and safe abortion and which are accessible, affordable, acceptable and convenient to all users.
2. All persons have the right to access to the widest possible range of safe, effective and acceptable methods of fertility regulation.
3. All persons have the right to be free to choose and to use a method of protection against unplanned pregnancy which is safe and acceptable to them.

The ninth is the right to health care and health protection (Article 25, Universal Declaration of Human Rights 1948). IPPF (2000) recognized the right as the enjoyment of the highest attainable standard of physical and mental health (IPPF 2000, 21–2).

1. All persons have the right to the highest possible quality in health care including all care related to their sexual and reproductive health.
2. All persons have the right to comprehensive health care services including access to all methods of fertility regulation including safe abortion and diagnosis and treatment for infertility and sexually transmitted diseases including Human Immunodeficiency Virus/Acquired Immune Deficiency Syndrome (HIV/AIDS).
3. All persons, and in particular the girl child and women, have the right to protection from traditional practices which are harmful to health.
4. All women have the right to pregnancy and infertility counseling which empowers them to make their own decisions, based on information impartially presented.
5. All persons have the right to sexual and reproductive health care services as part of primary health care, which are comprehensive, accessible, both

financially and geographically, private and confidential and which pay due regard to the dignity and comfort of that person.

6. All women have the right to appropriate services in connection with pregnancy, confinement and post-natal health care, as well as adequate nutrition during pregnancy and lactation.
7. All persons have the right to the protection of health, and safety in working conditions, including the safeguarding of the function of reproduction.
8. All working mothers have the right to be accorded paid maternity leave, or maternity leave with adequate social security benefits.
9. Every person has the right to sexual and reproductive health care including the following rights: information about benefits and risks of all fertility regulation methods; access to the widest range of services; choice to decide whether to use services, and which contraceptive method; safety concerning the methods and services made available; privacy when being offered information and services; confidentiality regarding personal information; dignity when using sexual and reproductive health care services; comfort concerning the equality of care of services offered; continuity guaranteeing future availability of services; and opinions about the service offered.

The right to the benefits of scientific progress and its applications is the tenth right (Article 27, Universal Declaration of Human Rights 1948). The right is indicated by the following rights with regard to women's reproductive rights (IPPF 2000, 23).

1. All persons shall have the benefit of and access to available reproductive health care technology, including that related to infertility, contraception and abortion, where to withhold access to such technology would have harmful effects on health and well-being.
2. All persons shall be entitled to protection from and information on any harmful effects of reproductive health care technology on their health and well-being.
3. All clients of sexual and reproductive health services have the right to access to all reproductive technologies which are safe and acceptable.

The right to freedom of assembly and political participation specified in the Universal Declaration of Human Rights (Article 20) is the number 11th right. The right is indicated by the following rights in relation to women's reproductive rights (IPPF 2000, 24).

1. All persons have the right to assemble and to canvass for sexual and reproductive health and rights.
2. All persons have the right to form an association which aims to promote sexual and reproductive health and well-being.

3. All persons have the right to seek to influence governments to place a priority on sexual and reproductive health and rights.

The last is the right to be free from torture and ill treatment (Article 5, Universal Declaration of Human Rights 1948). IPPF (2000) recognized the following rights as being related to women's reproductive rights.

1. All children have the right to protection from all forms of exploitation and, in particular, sexual exploitation, child prostitution and all forms of sexual abuse, assault, and harassment, including coercion of a child to engage in any unlawful sexual activity, the exploitation or use of children in prostitution or other unlawful sexual practices and the exploitative use of children in pornographic performances and materials.
2. No person should be subject to medical trials or experimentation related to sexuality or fertility regulation methods or techniques without their full, free and informed consent.
3. All women have the right to protection from traffic in women or exploitation of prostitution of them.
4. All civilians, women and men, have the right to be protected from degrading treatment and violence in relation to their sexuality and reproduction, especially during times of armed conflict.
5. All persons have the right to protection from rape, sexual assault, sexual abuse and sexual harassment. (pp. 25–6)

Appendix E
Developing Countries in Regional Aggregates

Arab States
(20 countries or areas)
Algeria, Bahrain, Djibouti, Egypt, Iraq, Jordan, Kuwait, Lebanon, Libya, Morocco, Occupied Palestinian Territories, Oman, Qatar, Saudi Arabia, Somalia, Sudan, Syrian Arab Republic, Tunisia, United Arab Emirates, Yemen.

East Asia and the Pacific
(28 countries or areas)
Brunei Darussalam, Cambodia, China, Fiji, Hong Kong, China (SAR), Indonesia, Kiribati, Korea (Democratic People's Republic of), Korea (Republic of), Lao People's Democratic Republic, Malaysia, Marshall Islands, Micronesia (Federated States of), Mongolia, Myanmar, Nauru, Palau, Papua New Guinea, Philippines, Samoa, Singapore, Solomon Islands, Thailand, Timor-Leste, Tonga, Tuvalu, Vanuatu, Viet Nam.

South Asia
(9 countries or areas)
Afghanistan, Bangladesh, Bhutan, India, Iran (Islamic Republic of), Maldives, Nepal, Pakistan, Sri Lanka.

Latin America and Caribbean
(33 countries or areas)
Antigua and Barbuda, Argentina, Bahamas, Barbados, Belize, Bolivia, Brazil, Chile, Colombia, Costa Rica, Cuba, Dominica, Dominican Republic, Ecuador, El Salvador, Grenada, Guatemala, Guyana, Haiti, Honduras, Jamaica, Mexico, Nicaragua, Panama, Paraguay, Peru, Saint Kitts and Nevis, Saint Lucia, Saint Vincent and the Grenadines, Suriname, Trinidad and Tobago, Uruguay, Venezuela (Bolivarian Republic of).

Southern Europe
(2 countries or areas)
Cyprus, Turkey.

Sub-Saharan Africa
(45 countries or areas)
Angola, Benin, Botswana, Burkina Faso, Burundi, Cameroon, Cape Verde, Central African Republic, Chad, Comoros, Congo, Congo (Democratic Republic of the), Côte d'Ivoire, Equatorial Guinea, Eritrea, Ethiopia, Gabon, Gambia, Ghana, Guinea, Guinea-Bissau, Kenya, Lesotho, Liberia, Madagascar, Malawi, Mali, Mauritania, Mauritius, Mozambique, Namibia, Niger, Nigeria, Rwanda, Sao Tome and Principe, Senegal, Seychelles, Sierra Leone, South Africa, Swaziland, Tanzania (United Republic of), Togo, Uganda, Zambia, Zimbabwe.

Source

United Nations Development Programme (UNDP). 2008. *Human Development Report 2007–2008*. (p. 392). Available at: http://hdr.undp.org/en/media/HDR_20072008_EN_complete.pdf.

Appendix F

Reproductive Health among Refugees and Internally Displaced Persons List of Selected Websites

Global Decade Report
www.rhrc.org/pdf/global_decade_report.pdf

Reproductive Health during Conflict and Displacement
www.who.int/reproductive-health/publications

Reproductive Health in Refugee Situation: An Inter-Agency Field Manual
www.who.int/disasters/tg.cfm?doctypeID=20

Reproductive Health of War-Affected Population: What Do We Know?
www.agi.usa.org/pubs/journals/2617400.html

Reproductive Health Outlook: Refugee Reproductive Health Section
www.rho.org/html/refugee_overview.htm

Reproductive Health Response in Conflict Consortium (formerly Reproductive Health for Refugees Consortium)
www.rhrc.org

Sexual and Gender-based Violence against Refugees, Returnees and Internally Displaced Persons: Guidelines for Prevention and Response
www.rhrc.org/pdf/gl_sgbv03.pdf.

State of the World's Mothers 2002: Mothers and Children in War and Conflict. Save the Children 2002
www.savethechildren.org/publications/mothers/2002/sowm2002.pdf

State of the Mothers 2003: Protecting Women and Children in War and Conflict. Save the Children 2003
www.planetwire/sowm-2003/sowm_2003.pdf

State of the World's Population 2000. Lives Together, Worlds Apart: Men and Women in a Time of Change
www.unfpa.org/swp/2000/english/ch02.html

Women's Commission for Refugee Women and Children.
www.womenscommission.org/index.html

Appendix G
Global Gag Rule Timeline

1973 January 22: Roe v. Wade: Abortion Legalized in the US

Roe v. Wade establishes, based on a constitutional right to privacy, a woman's right to seek an abortion in the United States. The full text of the Supreme Court's decision is available at: http://caselaw.lp.findlaw.com/scripts/getcase.pl?court=us&vol=410&invol=113. "Helms Amendment" Becomes Law: Later that year, Congress attached this amendment to the Foreign Assistance Act, sponsored by Senator Jesse Helms (R-NC), prohibiting the use of US foreign aid funds for abortion. The 1973 Helms Amendment is available at: http://www.usaid.gov/our_work/global_health/pop/restrictions.html.

1984 August: Mexico City Policy Introduced

At the International Conference on Population in Mexico City, the US delegation, headed by James Buckley, announced that the United States will no longer fund foreign, non-governmental organizations (NGOs) that provide, refer, counsel, or advocate for abortion. These restrictions were an executive branch policy in effect until 1993, but never became part of the permanent foreign assistance statute. It became known as the Mexico City Policy, and was later dubbed the "Global Gag Rule" by its opponents. The full text of the US government statement is available at: http://www.populationaction.org/Publications/Reports/Global_Gag_Rule_Restrictions/MexicoCityPolicy1984.pdf.

1985 IPPF De-funded

The US government suspended all support for the London-based International Planned Parenthood Federation (IPPF), because IPPF could not, by virtue of its constitution, comply with the global gag rule. At the time, IPPF was receiving roughly 25 percent of its budget from the United States; the defunding thus had serious financial implications.

US Government Sued Over Gag Rule

The DKT Memorial Fund launched the first of several legal challenges against the Global Gag Rule. This case was overturned in October 1989 by the US Court of Appeals for the District of Columbia, which ruled that the Global Gag Rule does not violate the constitutional rights to freedom of speech and association of US organizations by restricting their ability to work on abortion-related activities with foreign colleagues.DKT Memorial Fund v. US Agency for International Development (887 F.2d 275, 307–308).

1987 PPFA Sues USAID

Anticipating that its international program would be subjected to the global gag rule, Planned Parenthood Federation of America (PPFA) sued the United States Agency for International Development (USAID) in an attempt to reverse the policy.

The Supreme Court dismissed the case in September 1990, stating that PPFA's claim that the global gag rule violates the First Amendment right to free speech is unwarranted. Planned Parenthood Federation of America (PPFA), et al. versus US Agency for International Development, et al. (No. 90-1169) The full text of the Supreme Court's decision is available at: http://www.usdoj.gov/osg/briefs/1990/sg900226.txt.

1990 Pathfinder and Others Sue USAID

The Pathfinder Fund, the Population Council, and the Association for Voluntary Surgical Contraception sued USAID, claiming that the standard clause for AID eligibility under the global gag rule violates the constitutional rights of organizations like themselves to support abortion-related activities abroad. The US District Court in Washington D.C. later dismissed the case, ruling that the plaintiffs did not adequately substantiate their claim.

A deposition in the case by Duff Gillespie, Director of the USAID Office of Population, clarified USAID's interpretation of the global gag rule that still guided the implementation today. Pathfinder et al. v. USAID (746 F.Supp. 1992).

November: Impact of Global Gag Rule Studied

Investigators John Blane and Matthew Friedman released a report commissioned by USAID on the implementation of the Mexico City Policy in six countries: Bangladesh, Brazil, Egypt, Kenya, Pakistan, and Turkey. While Blane and Friedman concluded that most Cooperating Agencies and sub grantees (foreign NGOs) are complying with the policy, the fear of losing USAID funding has led to over-cautiousness concerning which activities are permitted under the Mexico City Policy. This caution has caused many foreign NGOs to avoid permitted activities for fear of losing funding. This fear and avoidance of permitted family planning activities highlights how the Mexico City Policy has a direct effect on access to reproductive health care and family planning services in developing countries, leaving women with fewer overall options.

1991 House Rejects Foreign Aid Authorization Bill

Conference report on the FY 1992-1993 Foreign Aid Authorization Bill (H.R. 2508 – H.Rept. 102-225), including language to reverse the global gag rule, was rejected by the House in a backlash against foreign aid in a time of domestic economic troubles.

The original text of the FY 1992-1993 Foreign Aid Authorization Bill, including Sec. 1204 – Family Planning Activities is available at: http://www.populationaction.org/Publications/Reports/Global_Gag_Rule_Restrictions/FY1992-3ForeignAidAuth.shtml.

1992 Congress Passes Aid Bill with Gag Rule Reversal Language

The FY 1992 Foreign Aid Appropriations Bill (H.Rept. 102-1011) includes language to reverse the Mexico City Policy, but was subsequently dropped following the threat of presidential veto from President George H.W. Bush.

1993 Mexico City Policy Repealed

As one of his first post-inauguration decisions, President Bill Clinton repealed the Mexico City Policy. In accordance with the Helms Amendment, however, NGOs must still maintain US funds in a segregated account, none of which may be used for abortion services. The Clinton's memorandum repealing the Mexico City Policy is available at: http://clinton6.nara.gov/1993/01/1993-01-22-aid-family-planning-grants-mexico-city-policy.html.

1996 Stalemate over Global Gag Rule

Congress did not impose any new policy restrictions in the FY97 foreign aid bill, but capped the funding level for bilateral population assistance at $385 million, and mandated that these funds not become available until March 1, 1997, six months into the fiscal year. These funds were subsequently metered out at a rate of 8 percent of the total over the following 12 and a half months.

In February, the House voted 220 to 209 and the Senate voted 53 to 45 to release family planning funds that had been blocked to punish President Clinton and congressional family planning supporters from both parties for refusing to accept the global gag rule.

1999 Fall: Congress Imposes Modified Global Gag Rule

To reach agreement on the payment of nearly $1 billion in US back dues to the United Nations, President Clinton and the House Republican leadership agreed to impose a modified global gag rule. The President was allowed to partially waive enforcement, but only on $15 million of total overseas family planning funding and at the cost of a $12.5 million funding cut.

2000 Fall: Population Funding Delayed on Election Outcome Gamble

While the FY 2001 Foreign Operations Appropriations Act does not reinstate the Mexico City Policy, it includes provisions which delayed USAID from obligating any funds until February 15, 2001. Republican and Democratic members of the Appropriations Committee gambled on the outcome of the election, effectively giving the new president the power to determine the future of US population assistance policy once in office.

2001 January 22: Bush Reinstates Global Gag Rule

President George W. Bush marked the 28th anniversary of Roe v. Wade by reinstating the Mexico City Policy via an executive memorandum, one of his first official acts as the 43rd president of the United States. Under the reinstated 'global gag rule,' post-abortion care would still be available through USAID-funded programs. President Bush's memorandum reinstating the Mexico City Policy is available at: http://www.whitehouse.gov/news/releases/20010123-5.html.

The White House Press Secretary's statement reiterating the President's support for family planning and post-abortion care is available at: http://www.whitehouse.gov/news/releases/20010123.html.

The full text of the original 1984 Mexico City Policy statement is available at: http://www.populationaction.org/Publications/Reports/Global_Gag_Rule_Restrictions/MexicoCityPolicy1984.pdf.

February: Global Democracy Promotion Act Introduced

In response to President Bush's reinstatement of the global gag rule, Representative Nita Lowey (D-NY) introduced the Global Democracy Promotion Act of 2001 in the House (H.R. 755.); while Senator Barbara Boxer (D-CA) introduced the same language in the Senate (S.367). The bill would effectively repeal the global gag rule, allowing disbursal of USAID funds to NGOs that counsel, refer, or advocate on behalf of abortion. The bi-partisan bills were co-sponsored by 31 senators and 71 representatives.

The text of the Global Democracy Promotion Act of 2001 is available at: http://frwebgate.access.gpo.gov/cgi-bin/getdoc.cgi?dbname=107_cong_bills&docid=f:s367rs.txt.pdf (Senate Version).

March 28: Bush Issues Presidential Memorandum Restoring Mexico City, Clarifying Stance on Post-Abortion Care

In response to increased agitation in the Congress against the reinstatement of the global gag rule, President Bush signed an executive memorandum, preventing Congress from challenging the policy under the 1996 Congressional Review Act. In addition, the memorandum clarified that USAID funding may be used to treat women following both legal and illegal abortions, although necessary equipment for such care may not be purchased with USAID funds.

The president's memorandum to the Acting Administrator of USAID, detailing the provisions of the global gag rule is available at: http://www.usaid.gov/business/business_opportunities/cib/pdf/cib0108r.pdf.

May: Global Gag Rule Challenge Survives Committees, But Fails in the House

On May 2, 2001, the House International Relations Committee voted to include provisions of the Global Democracy Promotion Act as an amendment to Foreign Relations Authorization Act, Fiscal Years 2002 and 2003 (H.R. 1646). This amendment was sponsored by Congresswoman Barbara Lee (D-CA).

The Foreign Relations Authorization Act, Fiscal Years 2002 and 2003 is available at: http://www.populationaction.org/Publications/Reports/Global_Gag_Rule_Restrictions/FY2002-3hr1646.shtml.

The White House's reaction to the Foreign Relations Authorization Act, Fiscal Years 2002 and 2003 is available at: http://www.whitehouse.gov/omb/legislative/sap/107-1/HR1646-r.html.

Later that month (May 17, 2001), the full House of Representatives, led by Rep. Henry Hyde (R-IL) and Rep. Chris Smith (R-NJ), struck the Lee Amendment with a vote of 218-210, effectively ensuring the continuance of the global gag rule.

The PAI's response to the stripping of the Global Democracy Promotion Act from the Foreign Relations Authorization Act is available at: http://www.populationaction.org/Press_Room/Viewpoints_and_Statements/2001/Remove_the_Gag!_PAI_Condemns_House_Vote_to_Uphold_the_Global_Gag_Rule.shtml.

In the Senate, the Global Democracy Promotion Act passed the Senate Foreign Relations Committee in a 12-7 vote on August 1, but the bill was never scheduled for consideration by the full Senate.

The PAI press release concerning the vote and foreign aid bill is available at: http://www.populationaction.org/Press_Room/Viewpoints_and_Statements/2000/Push_in_Congress_to_complete_foreign_aid_bill.shtml.

June: Advocacy Group Sues President Bush

On June 6, 2001, the Center for Reproductive Law and Policy (CRLP) launched a lawsuit against President George W. Bush, claiming that, "The global gag rule is global censorship that violates fairness, freedom, and democracy" in denying First Amendment rights to American lawyers working abroad with foreign partners.

The New York federal court dismissed CRLP's suit on July 31, 2001, claiming that CRLP lacked the standing to challenge the President and that any censorship that is taking place is voluntary since accepting USAID funds is a voluntary process. CRLP appealed to the US Court of Appeals for the Second Circuit.

A year later, on September 13, 2002, the US Court of Appeals for the Second Circuit also dismissed CRLP v. Bush, citing Planned Parenthood Federation of America, Inc. v. Agency for International Development, 915 F.2d 59 (2d. Cir. 1990) wherein it was determined that the global gag rule does not violate the First Amendment right to free speech since the decision to accept USAID funding is based on "independent choice."

September: USAID Affirms Support for Post-Abortion Care

Dr Duff Gillespie, the Deputy Assistant Administrator of the Population, Health, and Nutrition Center at USAID, released a "Dear Colleague" letter reminding field offices, Cooperating Agencies and USAID-sponsored programs of the importance and permissibility of post-abortion care under the global gag rule.

Dr Gillespie's letter is available at: http://www.usaid.gov/our_work/global_health/pop/mcpolicy_memo.pdf.

October: Senate Approves Language Overturning Gag Rule

The US Senate approved language overturning the global gag rule in the $15.5 billion FY 2002 Foreign Operations Appropriations Act. Based on this language, taken from the Global Democracy Promotion Act, the President was prohibited from refusing to fund foreign NGOs solely because they provide medical services, including counseling and referral, that are legal in their countries and are legal in the United States and prohibited from imposing free speech restrictions on foreign NGOs not imposed on US organizations receiving assistance under the foreign aid program.

2002 Fight for UNFPA Sidelines Gag Rule Battle

In January 2002, President Bush froze the $34 million US contribution to the United Nations Fund for Population Activities (UNFPA) approved by Congress in December 2001, at the behest of Rep. Chris Smith (R-NJ). Thus, throughout the FY03 budget process, Congressional supporters of international family planning focused on restoring UNFPA's funding, to the detriment of efforts to overturn the global gag rule.

Regrettably UNFPA's funding remained in limbo until July 22, 2002, when the State Department officially announced the revocation of its contribution. Although anti-gag rule language was included in the Senate version of the FY2003 Foreign Operations Bill, it did not survive the House-Senate conference negotiations and the final bill presented to the President was silent on the issue.

2003 February: White House Threatens Global Gag Rule Expansion

A policy shift contemplated by the White House was leaked by them to the press, alluding to a potential expansion of the Global Gag Rule to foreign non-governmental organizations (NGOs) receiving US funds for a broader but undefined set of reproductive health activities, including activities funded through the $15 billion initiative promised by President Bush for HIV/AIDS prevention and treatment. An exception would have been made for some foreign NGOs ineligible to receive family planning assistance under the gag rule, if they also implemented "discrete" HIV/AIDS projects.

March: African Officials and Health Professionals "Vehemently Oppose the Global Gag Rule."

Health professionals, lawyers, policymakers, non-governmental organizations, religious organizations and representatives of UNFPA, WHO and the World Bank came together in Addis Ababa, Ethiopia for the landmark "Action to Reduce Maternal Mortality in Africa" consultation on unsafe abortion. Participants resolve to reduce the impact and incidence of unsafe abortion, and called on African governments and the world community to oppose the Global Gag Rule.

The official communiqué is available at: http://www.populationaction.org/Publications/Reports/Global_Gag_Rule_Restrictions/UnsafeAbortionCommunique.pdf.

April: White House Withdraws Proposed Gag Rule Expansion to HIV/AIDS Funds

In a press briefing on the President's HIV/AIDS initiative, the White House made clear that the White House is "not expanding the Mexico City policy to cover this HIV-AIDS program." But there is nothing to prevent the President from changing his mind and extending the global gag rule through executive action at any time. The full transcript of the White House press briefing is available at: http://www.whitehouse.gov/news/releases/2003/04/20030429-3.html#12.

July: Senate Votes to Overturn Global Gag Rule

The Senate went on record in strong support of overturning the global gag rule when a "motion to table" (or "kill") an amendment to the State Department authorization bill (S. 925) offered by Senator Barbara Boxer (D-CA) was defeated on a vote of 43 to 53. Incorporating provisions of the Global Democracy Promotion Act, the Boxer amendment would prohibit the President from refusing to fund foreign NGOs solely because they provide medical services, including counseling and referral, that are legal in their countries and are legal in the United States and from imposing free speech restrictions on foreign NGOs not imposed on US organizations receiving assistance under the foreign aid program.

The Senate foreign policy bill was stalled, while the House-passed version did not address the global gag rule issue at all. President Bush announced his intention to veto the legislation if the final bill contained the Boxer amendment.

The veto threat is available at: http://www.whitehouse.gov/omb/legislative/sap/108-1/s925sap-s.pdf.

The PAI's statement on the vote is available at: http://www.populationaction.org/Press_Room/Press_Releases/2003/The_Gag_Must_Go!_PAI_Applauds_Senate_Vote_to_Overturn_Global_Gag_Rule.shtml.

The Congressional Record transcript of the debate over this amendment is available at: http://frwebgate.access.gpo.gov/cgi-in/getpage.cgi?dbname=2003_record&page=S9095&position=all.

August: Bush Extends Global Gag Rule to State Department

President Bush issued a memorandum to the Secretary of State directing that, in addition to international family planning funds channeled through USAID, the Global Gag Rule also applies to "family planning grants" awarded by the Department of State. At this point, it appeared this extension of the rule would primarily affect refugee reproductive health activities, unless the implementation of the policy was dramatically expanded beyond the interpretation of the restrictions used by USAID historically. The memorandum specifically exempts multilateral organizations and HIV/AIDS activities.

The memorandum is available at: http://www.whitehouse.gov/news/releases/2003/08/20030829-3.html.

October: Senate Passes Foreign Operations Bill with Amendment Overturning the Global Gag Rule

The Senate version of the foreign operations appropriations bill passed, with language similar to that attached by Senator Boxer to the State Department authorization bill in July. This language would prohibit the President from refusing to fund foreign NGOs solely because they provide medical services, including counseling and referral, that are legal in their countries and are legal in the United

States and from imposing free speech restrictions on foreign NGOs not imposed on US organizations receiving assistance under the foreign aid program.

The bill headed next to conference, where differences between the House and Senate versions of the bill would be negotiated. The House version does not mention the Global Gag Rule.

2004 January: President Bush Signs Omnibus Spending Bill without Language Overturning the Global Gag Rule

On January 23, President Bush signed the FY 2004 consolidated appropriation act. The bill does not contain language overturning the Global Gag Rule, which was inserted in the foreign operations section of the bill by the Senate in the fall of 2003, but later dropped during a House-Senate conference committee in November.

The previous day, the third anniversary of his reinstitution of the Global Gag Rule, the President touted his efforts in the international arena during a telephone address to anti-choice marchers protesting the 1973 Roe v. Wade Supreme Court decision, stating that "working with the Congress, we have refused the spend taxpayers' money on international programs that promote abortion overseas."

The transcript of the President's remarks to the "March for Life" is available at: http://www.whitehouse.gov/news/releases/2004/01/20040122-3.html.

The full text of consolidated appropriations act (H. Rpt. 108-401) is available at: http://thomas.loc.gov/cgi-bin/cpquery/T?&report=hr401&dbname=cp108&.

Autumn: Countdown 2015 Conference Examines Progress since the Cairo Conference, Sparking Renewed Media Interest in Global Gag Rule

Hundreds of government officials, public health experts and activists from around the world met in London to mark the tenth anniversary of the International Conference on Population and Development (ICPD) and to take stock of progress toward achieving the goals established in the ICPD Programme of Action. Media in the United States and abroad re-examined the ramifications of the Global Gag Rule on family planning and reproductive health clinics and providers in developing countries.

September: Senate Appropriations Committee Reinforces Policy that HIV/AIDS Programs Exempted from Global Gag Rule

Report language accompanying the FY 2005 foreign operations appropriations bill (S. 2812) approved by the Senate directs the State Department's Global AIDS Coordinator and the USAID Administrator to communicate to all relevant federal agencies that the Global Gag Rule restrictions do not apply to US HIV/AIDS assistance.

The full text of the Senate report (S. Rpt. 108-346) is available at: http://frwebgate.access.gpo.gov/cgi-bin/getdoc.cgi dbname=108_cong_reports&docid=f:sr346.108.pdf.

December: Final Spending Bill Again Leaves Global Gag Rule Restrictions Intact

On December 8, President Bush signed the FY 2005 consolidated appropriations act. As in the previous three years, the bill does not contain language overturning the Global Gag Rule, which had been incorporated in the Senate version of the foreign aid bill. Also dropped was a Senate amendment that waived restrictions on family planning, HIV/AIDS, and child survival programs if the policies (e.g. the Global Gag Rule) prevented efforts to "expand the availability and use of condoms for HIV/AIDS prevention and of contraceptives to reduce the incidence of abortion."

The full text of the Senate bill (S. 2812) is available at: http://frwebgate.access.gpo.gov/cgi-bin/getdoc.cgi?dbname=108_cong_bills&docid=f:s2812pcs.txt.pdf.

An index to the full text of the consolidated appropriations act (H. Rpt. 108-792) is available at: http://thomas.loc.gov/home/omni2005/index.htm.

2005 April: Senate votes to overturn Global Gag Rule

By a vote of 52-46, the Senate approved an amendment offered by Senators Barbara Boxer (D-CA) and Olympia Snowe (R-ME) to the State Department authorization bill (S. 600). Incorporating provisions of the Global Democracy Promotion Act, the Boxer amendment would prohibit the President from refusing to fund foreign NGOs solely because they provide medical services, including counseling and referral, that are legal in their countries and are legal in the United States and from imposing free speech restrictions on foreign NGOs not imposed on US organizations receiving assistance under the foreign aid program.

By the end of the year, the Senate had not completed action on the bill, and the House version of the bill, approved in July, did not include any language on the gag rule.

November: Amendment Exempting Contraceptives and Condoms from Global Gag Rule Dropped

During a House-Senate conference committee appointed to resolve differences between each chamber's respective version of the foreign operations appropriations bill, negotiators dropped a Senate-approved amendment stating that restrictions on family planning assistance – most notably the Global Gag Rule – should not be restrict efforts to expand access to condoms for HIV/AIDS prevention and of contraceptives to reduce the incidence of abortion.

Such a provision has been included by the Senate for several years and has been similarly dropped. President Bush signed the final bill without the Senate amendment (H.R. 3057) on November 14.

November/December: Global Gag Rule Not Extended to HIV/AIDS Assistance

An announcement of a request for application (RFA) for a five-year, $193 million integrated health project in Kenya triggered concerns that the gag rule had been extended to US HIV/AIDS assistance. This was not the case. The RFA was for an integrated HIV/AIDS and reproductive health care project funded by both HIV/AIDS and family planning funds, and it was riddled with errors. The USAID/Kenya mission withdrew the RFA and reissued a corrected version in December maintaining the integrated nature of the project while clarifying that foreign NGOs receiving only HIV/AIDS assistance are exempt from the gag rule.

The global gag rule continued to apply to US family planning assistance. However, a presidential memorandum issued in August 2003 specifically clarified that HIV/AIDS assistance is exempt from the gag rule (link). Correspondence from Ambassador Randall Tobias, Office of the Global AIDS Coordinator, and Kent Hill, Assistant Administrator for Global Health, USAID, reiterated that the gag rule does not apply to HIV/AIDS assistance.

2006 June: Senate Appropriations Committee Endorses Full Repeal of Global Gag Rule

During full committee markup, Senate appropriators approved an amendment to its version of the FY 2007 State-Foreign Operations Appropriations bill that overturns the Global Gag Rule, an executive branch policy, by prohibiting the President from refusing to fund foreign organizations solely because they provide medical services, including counseling and referral, that are legal in their countries and are legal in the United States and from imposing free speech restrictions on foreign NGOs not imposed on US organizations receiving assistance under the foreign aid program. (The House version of bill, also passed in full committee in June, did not contain a repeal provision.) The Senate language was dropped when Congress sent a long-term continuing resolution to keep the government funded to the President for his signature in February 2007.

2007 June: House Votes to Grant Exemption from the Global Gag Rule for Contraceptive Supplies

On a vote of 223-201, the House adopted an amendment to the FY 2008 State-Foreign Operations Appropriations bill (H.R. 2764) inserted by Rep. Nita Lowey, the chair of the subcommittee with jurisdiction over the legislation, exempting overseas NGO family planning providers from the restrictions of the Gag Rule that cuts off the flow of US-donated contraceptives and condoms. Under this provision, providers that have refused to abide by the terms of the Gag Rule would be eligible to receive contraceptives from the US government. Family planning opponents were unsuccessful in their efforts to strike the Lowey amendment from the House bill, specifically when an amendment by Reps. Chris Smith (R-NJ) and Bart Stupak (D-MI) to delete the contraceptives exemption was rejected on a vote of 205 to 218. This was the first time that family planning advocates have won a clear-cut victory on an anti-Gag Rule amendment in the House since 1991.

Roll call vote on the Lowey amendment is available at: http://clerk.house.gov/evs/2007/roll533.xml.

Roll call vote on the Smith-Stupak amendment is available at: http://clerk.house.gov/evs/2007/roll534.xml.

September: Senate Overturns Global Gag Rule in its Entirety and Passes Contraceptive Exemption

During its debate of the FY 2008 State-foreign ops bill, the Senate not only adopted a contraceptive exemption from the Gag Rule but went a step further and voted to repeal the Gag Rule entirely. The Senate vote marks the first time since the Gag Rule has been in force – from 1984 to 1993 and again since 2001 – that both the House and Senate have passed legislation to repeal or modify the restriction that has wreaked havoc on family planning efforts, especially in Africa.

On a vote of 53 to 41, the Senate approved a bipartisan pro-family planning amendment authored by Senators Barbara Boxer (D-CA) and Olympia Snowe (R-ME) that overturns the Gag Rule, an executive branch policy, by prohibiting the President from refusing to fund foreign organizations solely because they provide medical services, including counseling and referral, that are legal in their countries and are legal in the United States and from imposing free speech restrictions on foreign NGOs not imposed on US organizations receiving assistance under the foreign aid program.

An anti-family planning amendment offered by Sen. Sam Brownback (R-KS) that proposed striking the language incorporated in both the House and Senate bills expanding access to contraceptives by providing a limited exemption from the Gag Rule solely for USAID-donated contraceptives for foreign organizations otherwise ineligible for US family planning assistance because of the Gag Rule was soundly rejected on a vote 41 to 53.

Roll call vote on the Boxer-Snowe amendment is available at: http://www.senate.gov/legislative/LIS/roll_call_lists/roll_call_vote_cfm.cfm?congress=110&session=1&vote=00319.

Roll call vote on the Brownback amendment is available at: http://www.senate.gov/legislative/LIS/roll_call_lists/roll_call_vote_cfm.cfm?congress=110&session=1&vote=00320.

December: Amendment Exempting Contraceptives from Global Gag Rule in Veto Showdown

Although both the House and Senate adopted a contraceptive exemption to the Gag Rule – the first time both houses had repudiated this harmful policy in the same year since its imposition in 1984 – the amendment was not enacted into law. Despite the fact both the House and Senate-passed bills contained an identical contraceptive exemption amendment, the provision was dropped during the House-Senate conference on the omnibus spending bill in the face of a veto threat by President Bush.

2008 July: Senate Committee Again Goes on Record for Repeal of Global Gag Rule

When the Senate Appropriations Committee adopted a full repeal of the Global Gag Rule during full committee markup of the FY 2009 State-Foreign Operations Appropriations bill, Senate family planning supporters continued to register their opposition to this harmful presidential policy. (The House version of the bill is silent on the topic.) Final action on most of the FY 2009 appropriations bills was deferred until after the 2008 presidential and congressional elections, and funding for foreign aid programs remained part of a long-term continuing resolution at the end of 2008.

August: Democratic Party Platform Endorses Gag Rule Repeal

During the Democratic National Convention in Denver, delegates approved a party platform that states: "We will repeal the global gag rule and reinstate funding to the United Nations Population Fund (UNFPA). We will expand access to health care and nutrition for women and reduce the burden of maternal mortality."

The Democratic Party platform is available at: http://www.democrats.org/a/party/platform.html.

2009 January: President Obama Rescinds Global Gag Rule

On January 23rd, President Obama rescinded the Global Gag Rule by issuing a presidential memorandum to the Secretary of State and USAID Administrator directing that the gag rule restrictions be excluded from all future USAID and State Department assistance awards and that the restrictions be removed from all current family planning grants and assistance agreements as soon as possible. In issuing the memorandum, President Obama released a statement that called the Global Gag Rule "unnecessarily broad and unwarranted" and noted that it had "undermined efforts to promote safe and effective voluntary family planning in

developing countries." He called for an "end to the politicization of this issue" and announced that his administration would "initiate a fresh conversation on family planning, working to find areas of common ground" and would "reach out to those on all sides of this issue to achieve the goal of reducing unintended pregnancies." In rescinding the Global Gag Rule, President Obama also announced his intention to work with Congress to restore a US contribution to the United Nations Population Fund, pending the completion of the FY 2009 appropriations process.
President Obama's memorandum to the Secretary of State and the USAID Administrator rescinding the Global Gag Rule is available at: http://www.whitehouse.gov/the_press_office/MexicoCityPolicy-VoluntaryPopulationPlanning/.

President Obama's statement in rescinding the Global Gag Rule is available at: http://www.whitehouse.gov/statement-released-after-the-president-rescinds/.

Senate Rejects Amendment to Re-impose the Global Gag Rule Legislatively

On January 28th, just five days after President Obama repealed it, the Senate resoundingly defeated a surprise amendment to an unrelated children's health insurance bill (H.R. 2), offered by Senator Mel Martinez (R-FL), to restore the Global Gag Rule by nullifying the January 23rd presidential memorandum and by prohibiting US family planning assistance to "any private, non-governmental, or multilateral organization that performs or actively promotes abortion as a method of birth control." The amendment failed on a vote of 37 for and 60 against (the pro-family planning position). The Martinez amendment not only would have reimposed the Global Gag Rule on foreign NGOs, it sought to expand the reach of the restriction on eligibility to receive US family planning assistance to US-based organizations and multilateral organizations.

Roll call vote on the Martinez amendment is available at: http://www.senate.gov/legislative/LIS/roll_call_lists/roll_call_vote_cfm.cfm?congress=111&session=1&vote=00019.

The Congressional Record transcript of the debate over this amendment is available at: http://frwebgate.access.gpo.gov/cgi-bin/getpage.cgi?position=all&page=S955&dbname=2009_record.

Source

Population Action International (PAI). 2009. Available at: www.populationaction.org/issues/US_Policies_and_funding/global_gag_rule.shml.

Appendix H
President Obama's Memorandum (January 23, 2009)

MEMORANDUM FOR THE SECRETARY OF STATE
THE ADMINISTRATOR OF THE UNITED STATES AGENCY FOR INTERNATIONAL DEVELOPMENT

SUBJECT: Mexico City Policy and Assistance for Voluntary Population Planning

The Foreign Assistance Act of 1961 (22 USC. 2151b(f)(1)), prohibits non-governmental organizations (NGOs) that receive Federal funds from using those funds "to pay for the performance of abortions as a method of family planning, or to motivate or coerce any person to practice abortions." The August 1984 announcement by President Reagan of what has become known as the "Mexico City Policy" directed the United States Agency for International Development (USAID) to expand this limitation and withhold USAID funds from NGOs that use non-USAID funds to engage in a wide range of activities, including providing advice, counseling, or information regarding abortion, or lobbying a foreign government to legalize or make abortion available. The Mexico City Policy was in effect from 1985 until 1993, when it was rescinded by President Clinton. President George W. Bush reinstated the policy in 2001, implementing it through conditions in USAID grant awards, and subsequently extended the policy to "voluntary population planning" assistance provided by the Department of State.

These excessively broad conditions on grants and assistance awards are unwarranted. Moreover, they have undermined efforts to promote safe and effective voluntary family planning programs in foreign nations. Accordingly, I hereby revoke the Presidential memorandum of January 22, 2001, for the Administrator of USAID (Restoration of the Mexico City Policy), the Presidential memorandum of March 28, 2001, for the Administrator of USAID (Restoration of the Mexico City Policy), and the Presidential memorandum of August 29, 2003, for the Secretary of State (Assistance for Voluntary Population Planning). In addition, I direct the Secretary of State and the Administrator of USAID to take the following actions with respect to conditions in voluntary population planning assistance and USAID grants that were imposed pursuant to either the 2001 or 2003 memoranda and that are not required by the Foreign Assistance Act or any other law: (1) immediately waive such conditions in any current grants, and (2) notify current grantees, as soon as possible, that these conditions have been waived. I further direct that the Department of State and USAID immediately cease imposing these conditions in any future grants.

This memorandum is not intended to, and does not, create any right or benefit, substantive or procedural, enforceable at law or in equity by any party against the United States, its departments, agencies, or entities, its officers, employees, or agents, or any other person.

The Secretary of State is authorized and directed to publish this memorandum in the *Federal Register*.

BARACK OBAMA
THE WHITE HOUSE, January 23, 2009.

Source

The White House, United States. 2009. Available at: www.whitehouse.gov/the_press_office/MexicoCityPolicy-VoluntaryPopulationPlanning.

REPEAL OF THE MEXICO CITY POLICY
HILLARY RODHAM CLINTON SECRETARY OF STATE
Statement upon the repeal of the Mexico City Policy by President Obama
Washington, DC

President Obama's repeal of the Global Gag Rule, which has prevented women around the world from gaining access to essential information and healthcare services, is a welcomed and important step taken during the first days of the Administration.

For the past seven years, this policy has made it more difficult for women around the world to gain access to essential information and healthcare services. Rather than limiting women's ability to receive reproductive health services, we should be supporting programs that help women and their partners make decisions to ensure their health and the health of their families.

As I said in Beijing at the United Nations 4th World Conference on Women, women must not be denied the right to plan their own families. I look forward to working with the President, my colleagues in the Administration, and the NGO community to promote programs and policies that ensure women and girls have full access to health information and services.

Source

The White House, United States. 2009. Available at: www.whitehouse.gov/the_press_office/MexicoCityPolicy-VoluntaryPopulationPlanning.

Appendix I
List of Selected Non-governmental Organizations (NGOs) Women's Reproductive Health and Reproductive Rights

Action Health Incorporated
www.actionhealthinc.org

Adolescent Reproductive Health Network
www.argne.org

Africa Regional Sexuality Resource Centre
www.arsrc.org

African Partnership for Sexual and Reproductive Health and Rights of Women (AMANITARE) www.amanitare.org

African Women's Development Fund (AWDF)
www.awdf.org

(The) Alan Guttmacher Institute (AGI)
www.agi-usa.org

Amnesty International (AI) – Stop Violence against Women Campaign
http://web.amnesty.org/actforwomen/indexpeng

Asian Communities for Reproductive Justice (ACRJ)
www.acrj.org

AVSC International
www.avsc.org

(The) Bill and Melinda Gates Foundation
www.gatesfoundation.org

Center for African Family Studies (CAFS)
www.cafs,org

Center for AIDS Prevention Studies (CAPS)
www.caps.ucsf.edu

Center for Development and Population Activities. (CEDPA)
www.cedpa.org

Center for Health and Gender Equity (CHANGE)
www.genderhealth.org

Center for Reproductive Rights (CRR)
www.reproductiverights.org

Center for Reproductive Law and Policy (CRLP)
www.crlp.org

Center for the Study of AIDS in South Africa (CSA)
www.csa.za.org

Centers for Diseases Control and Prevention (CDC)
www.cdc.org

Centre for African Studies (CAFS)
www.cafs.org

Centre for the AIDS Program of Research in South Africa (CAPRISA)
www.caprisa.org

Coalition for Research in Women's Health (CRWH)
www.crwh.org

Council on Health Research for Development (Supporting national health research in low and middle income countries)
www.cohred.ch

Development Gateway HIV/AIDS
http://topics.developmentgateway.org/hiv

Doctors of the World (DOW)
www.healthright.org

Duke University Library, NGOs – Women in Development
http://library.duke.edu/research/subject/guides/ngo_guide/ngo_links/women.html

EC/UNFPA Initiative for Reproductive Health in Asia
www.asia-initiative.org

Eldis Gender and HIV/AIDS Dossier
www.eldis.org/gender/dossiers

Electronic Articles on Adolescent Reproductive and Sexual Health
www.unescobkk.org/ips/arh-web

Family Care International
www.familycareintl.org

Family Health International (FHI)
www.fhi.org/en/index.htm

Federation for International Cooperation of Health Services and Systems Research Centers (IFRC)
www.ifrc.org

Foundation for Women's Health, Research and Development UK (Forward Foundation) (A leading voluntary organization in the UK working toward elimination of FGM world)
www.forwarduk.org.uk

Global Action Network
www.globalactionnetwork.org

Global Forum for Health Research
www.globalforumhealth.org

Global Fund for Women
www.globalfundforwomen.org

Global Fund to Fight AIDS, Tuberculosis and Malaria (GFATM)
www.theglobalfund.org/en

Global Health Council
www.globalhealth.org

Global Reproductive Health Forum, Harvard University (GRHF)
www.hsph.harvard.edu/grhf

Harvard Center for Population and Development Studies (HCPDS), Harvard School of Public Health
www.hsph.harvard.edu/centers-institutes/population-development

Health Action Information Network (HAIN)
www.hain.org

Health and Development Networks (HDN)
www.hdnet.org/home.asp

Harvard FXB Center for Health and Human Rights
www.hsph.harvard.edu/fxbcenter

Human Rights Watch
www.hrw.org

Interact Worldwide
www.interactworldwide.org

International Alliance of Women
www.tiaw.org

International Association for Adolescent Health (IAAH)
www.iaah.org

International Association for Maternal and Neonatal Health
www.gfmer.ch/000_iamaneh.htm

International Bureau for Children's Rights (IBCR)
www.ibcr.org

International Center for AIDS Care and Treatment Programs (ICAP)
www.icap.org

International Center for Reproductive Health (ICRH)
www.icrh.org

International Center for Research on Women (ICRW)
www.icrw.org/html/issues/violence.htm

International Council of Women (ICW)
www.icw-cif.org

International Council on Management of Population Programmes (ICOMP)
www.icomp.org

International Federation of Fertility Societies (IFFA)
www.iffa-reproduction.org

International HIV/AIDS Alliance
www.aidsalliance.org

International Organization for Women and Development (IOWD)
www.iowd.org

International Planned Parenthood Federation (IPPF)
www.ippf.org

International Union against Sexually Transmitted Infections (IUSTI)
www.iusti.org

International Union for the Scientific Study of Population (IUSSP)
www.iussp.org

International Women's Health Coalition (IWHC)
www.iwhc.org

(The) Latin American and Caribbean Women's Health Network (LACWHN)
www.lacwhn.org

Pan American Health Organization
http://new.paho.org

Pathfinder International
www.pathfind.org

Population Action International (PAI)
www.populationaction.org

(The) Population Council
www.popcouncil.org

(The) Population Resource Center (PRC)
www.prc.org

Population Services International (PSI)
www.psi.org

Project HOPE
www.projecthope.org

Refugee Studies Center at Oxford University
www.rsc.ox.ac.uk

Reproductive Health for Refugees Consortium (RHRC)
www.rhrc.org

Save the Children Fund
www.savethechildren.org

(The) Support for Analysis and Research in Africa (SARA)
www.sara.org

UNIFEM Gender and HIV/AIDS Web Portal: Violence against Women and HIV/AIDS
www.genderandaids.org/modules.php?name=News&new_topic=9

United Nations Development Programme (UNDP)
www.undp.org

United Nations Children's Fund (UNICEF).
www.unicef.org

United Nations Development Fund for Women (UNIFEM)
www.unifem.org

United Nations Fund for Population Activities (UNFPA)
www.unfpa.org

United Nations Fund for Population Activities (UNFPA) – Violence against Women: A Public Health Priority
www.unfpa.org/intercenter/violence

United Nations High Commissioner for Refugees (UNHCR)
www.unhcr.org

United Nations Joint Programme on HIV/AIDS (UNAIDS)
www.unaids.org

United Nations Population Information Network (POPIN)
www.popin.org

(The) William J. Clinton Foundation
www.clintonfoundation.org

Women, Children and HIV Resources for Prevention and Treatment
www.womenchildrenhiv.org

Women Watch, United Nations
www.un.org/womenwatch

Women's Commission for Refugee Women and Children (WCRWC)
www.wcrwc.org

Women's Refugee Commission
www.womensrefugeecommission.org

World Bank, Improving Reproductive Health: The Role of the World Bank
www.worldbank.org/extdr/hnp/population/imp_rh

World Health Organization – Department of Gender and Women's Health
www.who.int/gender/en

World Health Organization – Initiative on HIV/AIDS and Sexually Transmitted Infections (HSI) www.icomp.org.my/South-South/rhweb/rhweb54.htm

World Health Organization – Sexual Violence Research Initiative
www.who.int/gender/violence/sexviolresearch/en

World Health Organization – Statistical Information System (WHOSIS)
www.who.int/whosis/en

World Health Organization Violence against Women and HIV/AIDS
www.who.int/gender/violence/vawandhiv/en

World YWCA HIV/AIDS
www.worldywca.org/aids/index.html

Appendix J
Countries in Major World Aggregates

Developing Countries
(137 countries or areas)

Afghanistan, Algeria, Angola, Antigua and Barbuda, Argentina, Bahamas, Bahrain, Bangladesh, Barbados, Belize, Benin, Bhutan, Bolivia, Botswana, Brazil, Brunei Darussalam, Burkina Faso, Burundi, Cambodia, Cameroon, Cape Verde, Central African Republic, Chad, Chile, China, Colombia, Comoros, Congo, Congo (Dem. Rep. of the), Costa Rica, Côte d'Ivoire, Cuba, Cyprus, Djibouti, Dominica, Dominican Republic, Ecuador, Egypt, El Salvador, Equatorial Guinea, Eritrea, Ethiopia, Fiji, Gabon, Gambia, Ghana, Grenada, Guatemala, Guinea, Guinea-Bissau, Guyana, Haiti, Honduras, Hong Kong, China (SAR), India, Indonesia, Iran (Islamic Republic of), Iraq, Jamaica, Jordan, Kenya, Kiribati, Korea (Democratic People's Republic of), Korea (Republic of), Kuwait, Lao People's Democratic Republic, Lebanon, Lesotho, Liberia, Libya, Madagascar, Malawi, Malaysia, Maldives, Mali, Marshall Islands, Mauritania, Mauritius, Mexico, Micronesia (Federated States of), Mongolia, Morocco, Mozambique, Myanmar, Namibia, Nauru, Nepal, Nicaragua, Niger, Nigeria, Occupied Palestinian Territories, Oman, Pakistan, Palau, Panama, Papua New Guinea, Paraguay, Peru, Philippines, Qatar, Rwanda, Saint Kitts and Nevis, Saint Lucia, Saint Vincent and the Grenadines, Samoa, Sao Tome and Principe, Saudi Arabia, Senegal, Seychelles, Sierra Leone, Singapore, Solomon Islands, Somalia, South Africa, Sri Lanka, Sudan, Suriname, Swaziland, Syrian Arab Republic, Tanzania (United Republic of), Thailand, Timor-Leste, Togo, Tonga, Trinidad and Tobago, Tunisia, Turkey, Tuvalu, Uganda, United Arab Emirates, Uruguay, Vanuatu, Venezuela (Bolivarian Republic of), Viet Nam, Yemen, Zambia, Zimbabwe.

Least Developed Countries (LDCs)
(50 countries or areas)

Afghanistan, Angola, Bangladesh, Benin, Bhutan, Burkina Faso, Burundi, Cambodia, Cape Verde, Central African Republic, Chad, Comoros, Congo (Democratic Republic of the), Djibouti, Equatorial Guinea, Eritrea, Ethiopia, Gambia, Guinea, Guinea-Bissau, Haiti, Kiribati, Lao People's Democratic Republic, Lesotho, Liberia, Madagascar, Malawi, Maldives, Mali, Mauritania, Mozambique, Myanmar, Nepal, Niger, Rwanda, Samoa, Sao Tome and Principe,

Senegal, Sierra Leone, Solomon Islands, Somalia, Sudan, Tanzania (United Republic of) Timor-Leste, Togo, Tuvalu, Uganda, Vanuatu, Yemen, Zambia.

Central and Eastern Europe and the Commonwealth of Independent States (CIS)
(28 countries or areas)

Albania, Armenia, Azerbaijan, Belarus, Bosnia and Herzegovina, Bulgaria, Croatia, Czech Republic, Estonia, Georgia, Hungary, Kazakhstan, Kyrgyzstan, Latvia, Lithuania, Macedonia (TFYR), Moldova, Montenegro, Poland, Romania, Russian Federation, Serbia, Slovakia, Slovenia, Tajikistan, Turkmenistan, Ukraine, Uzbekistan.

Organization for Economic Co-operation and Development (OECD)
(30 countries or areas)

Australia, Austria, Belgium, Canada, Czech Republic, Denmark, Finland, France, Germany, Greece, Hungary, Iceland, Ireland, Italy, Japan, Korea (Republic of), Luxembourg, Mexico, Netherlands, New Zealand, Norway, Poland, Portugal, Slovakia, Spain, Sweden, Switzerland, Turkey, United Kingdom, United States.

High-income OECD
(24 countries or areas)

Australia, Austria, Belgium, Canada, Denmark, Finland, France, Germany, Greece, Iceland, Ireland, Italy, Japan, Korea (Republic of), Luxembourg, Netherlands, New Zealand, Norway, Portugal, Spain, Sweden, Switzerland, United Kingdom, United States.

Source

United Nations Development Programme (UNDP). 2008. *Human Development Report 2007–2008*. (p. 376). Available at: http://hdr.undp.org/en/media/HDR_20072008_EN_complete.pdf.

Appendix K
Countries or Areas in Income Aggregates

High Income
(55 countries or areas)

Andorra, Antigua and Barbuda, Aruba, Australia, Austria, Bahamas, Bahrain, Belgium, Bermuda, Brunei Darussalam, Canada, Cayman Islands, Cyprus,Denmark,Faeroe Islands, Finland, France, French Polynesia, Germany, Greece, Greenland, Guam, Hong Kong China (SAR), Iceland, Ireland, Isle of Man, Israel, Italy, Japan, Korea (Republic of), Kuwait, Liechtenstein, Luxembourg, Macao China (SAR), Malta, Monaco, Netherlands, Netherlands Antilles, New Caledonia, New Zealand, Norway, Portugal, Puerto Rico, Qatar, San Marino, Saudi Arabia, Singapore, Slovenia, Spain, Sweden, Switzerland, United Arab Emirates, United Kingdom, United States, United States Virgin Islands.

Middle Income
(97 countries or areas)

Albania, Algeria, American Samoa, Angola, Argentina, Armenia, Azerbaijan, Barbados, Belarus, Belize, Bolivia, Bosnia and Herzegovina, Botswana, Brazil, Bulgaria, Cameroon, Cape Verde, Chile, China, Colombia, Congo, Costa Rica, Croatia, Cuba, Czech Republic, Djibouti, Dominica, Dominican Republic, Ecuador, Egypt, El Salvador, Equatorial Guinea, Estonia, Fiji, Gabon, Georgia, Grenada, Guatemala, Guyana, Honduras, Hungary, Indonesia, Iran (Islamic Republic of), Iraq, Jamaica, Jordan, Kazakhstan, Kiribati, Latvia, Lebanon, Lesotho, Libya Arab Jamahiriya, Lithuania, Macedonia (TFYR), Malaysia, Maldives, Marshall Islands, Mauritius, Mexico, Micronesia (Federated States of), Moldova, Montenegro, Morocco, Namibia, Nicaragua, Northern Mariana Islands, Occupied Palestinian Territories, Oman, Palau, Panama, Paraguay, Peru, Philippines, Poland, Romania, Russian Federation, Saint Kitts and Nevis, Saint Lucia, Saint Vincent and the Grenadines, Samoa, Serbia, Seychelles, Slovakia, South Africa, Sri Lanka, Suriname, Swaziland, Syrian Arab Republic, Thailand, Tonga, Tunisia, Turkey, Turkmenistan, Ukraine, Uruguay, Vanuatu, Venezuela (Bolivarian Republic of).

Low Income
(54 countries or areas)

Afghanistan, Bangladesh, Benin, Bhutan, Burkina Faso, Burundi, Cambodia, Central African Republic, Chad, Comoros, Congo (Democratic Republic of the), Côte d'Ivoire, Eritrea, Ethiopia, Gambia, Ghana, Guinea, Guinea-Bissau, Haiti, India, Kenya, Korea (Democratic People's Republic of), Kyrgyzstan, Lao People's Democratic Republic, Liberia, Madagascar, Malawi, Mali, Mauritania, Mongolia, Mozambique, Myanmar, Nepal, Niger, Nigeria, Pakistan, Papua New Guinea, Rwanda, Sao Tome and Principe, Senegal, Sierra Leone, Solomon Islands, Somalia, Sudan, Tajikistan, Tanzania (United Republic of), Timor-Leste, Togo, Uganda, Uzbekistan, Viet Nam, Yemen, Zambia, Zimbabwe.

Source

United Nations Development Programme (UNDP). 2008. *Human Development Report 2007-2008*. (p. 375). Available at: http://hdr.undp.org/en/media/HDR_20072008_EN_complete.pdf.

Bibliography

Acharya, M. 1979. *The Status of Women in Nepal, Volume 1: Background Report, Part 1, Statistical Profile of Nepalese Women: A Critical Review*. Kathmandu: Center for Economic Development and Administration.

Acharya, M. 1981. *The Status of Women in Nepal, Volume 2: Field Studies, Part 1, The Maithili Women of Sissia*. Kathmandu: Center for Economic Development and Administration.

Ackerly, B.A. 1995. Testing the tools of development: credit programmes, loan involvement, and women's empowerment. *IDS Bulletin*, 26 (3), 56–68.

Adler, N., Boyce, T., Chesney, M., Cohen, S., Folkman, S., Kahn, R. and Syme, L. 1994. Socioeconomic status and health: the challenge of the gradient. *American Psychologist*, 49, 15–24.

Ahmed-Ghosh, H. 2006.Voices of Afghan women. *International Feminist Journal of Politics*, 8 (1), 110–28.

Aitken, I. and Reichenbach, L. 1994. Reproductive and sexual health services: expanding access and enhancing quality, in *Population Policies Reconsidered: Health, Empowerment, and Rights,* edited by G. Sen, A. German, and L.C. Chen. Boston, MA: Harvard University Press, 177–92.

Allison, P.D. 1999. *Multiple Regression: A Primer*. Thousand Oaks, CA: Pine Forge Press.

Always, J. 1995. The trouble with gender: tales of the still-missing feminist revolution in sociological theory. *Sociological Theory*, 13 (3), 209–28.

Amnesty International. 2003. *Amnesty International Annual Report on Country Human Rights Practice 2003*. Available at: www.unca.edu/politicalscience/pts.xls.

Aminzade, R. 1993. *Ballots and Barricades: Class Formation and Republican Politics in France, 1830–1871*. Princeton, NJ: Princeton University Press.

Ankney, C.D. 1995. Sex differences in relative brain size: the mismeasure of women too? *Personality and Intelligence*, 16, 329–36.

Ashford, L.S. 2001. New population policies: advancing women's health and rights. *Population Bulletin,* 56 (1), 3–43.

Bangser, M. 2002. Policy environments, macroeconomics, programming, and participation, in *Engendering International Health: The Challenge of Equity*, edited by G. Sen, A. George, and P. Ostlin. Boston, MA: MIT Press, 257–80.

Bartram, J., Lewis, K., Lenton, R. and Wright, A. 2005. Focusing on improved water and sanitation of health. *The Lancet*, 365, 810–12.

Basu, A.M. 2000. Gender in population research: confusing implications for health policy. *Population Studies,* 54, 19–28.

Basu, A.M. and Koolwal, G. 2004. Two notions of female autonomy and their implications for reproductive health, in *A Focus on Gender: Collected Papers Using DHS Data*. Washington, DC: Macro International.

Becker, G.S. 1985. Human capital, effort, and the sexual division of labor. *Journal of Labor Economics,* 3, 33–58.

Bell, D. 2001. The coming of post-industrial society, in *Social Stratification: Class, Race, and Gender in Sociological Perspective*, edited by David B. Grusky. Boulder, CO: Westview Press, 805–17.

Bennett, T. 1997. Women's health in maternal and child health: time for a new tradition? *Maternal and Child Health Journal*, 1 (4), 253–65.

Bentham, J. 1780. *Introduction to the Principles of Morals and Legislation.* Available at: www.la.utexas.edu/research/poltheory/bentham/ipml/ipml.toc.htm.

Berkman, L.F. and Kawachi, I. 2000. *Social Epidemiology*. New York: Oxford University Press.

Berkovitch, N. 1999. *From Motherhood to Citizenship: Women's Rights and International Organizations.* Baltimore, MD: Johns Hopkins University Press.

Bertrand, J. and Tsui, A.1995. *Introduction: Indicators for Reproductive Health Program Evaluation.* Chapel Hill, NC: The Evaluation Project.

Bird, S.T. and Bauman, K.E. 1995. The relationship between structural and health services variables and state-level infant mortality in the United States. *American Journal of Public Health,* 85 (1), 26–32.

Birn, A. 1999. Skirting the issues: women and international health in historical perspective. *American Journal of Public Health,* 89 (3), 399–407.

Blanc, A.K. 2001. The effect of power in sexual relationships on sexual and reproductive health: an examination of evidence. *Studies in Family Planning*, 32 (3), 189–213.

Blanchard, K., Elul, B. and Rao, S.R. 1999. *Reproductive Health Indicators: Moving Forward.* Available at: www.popcouncil.org/pdfs/ebert/rhindicators.pdf.

Blane, J. and Friedman, M. 1990. *Mexico City Policy Implementation Stud*y. Population Technical Assistance Project Occasional Paper No. 5. Available at: http://pdf.usaid.gov/pdf_docs/PNABG765.pdf.

Blood, R.O., Jr and Wolfe, D.M. 1960. *Husbands and Wives: The Dynamics of Marriage Living*. New York: Free Press.

Bloom, S., Wypil, D. and Gupta, M.D. 2001. Dimensions of women's autonomy and the influence on maternal health care utilization in a north Indian city. *Demography*, 38 (1), 67–78.

Blumberg, R.L. 1984. A general theory of gender stratification, in *Sociological Theory*, edited by R. Collins. New York: Jossey-Bass.

Blumberg, R.L. 1989. Toward a feminist theory of development, in *Feminism and Sociological Theory*, edited by R. Wallace. Newbury Park, CA: Sage.

Bollen, K.A. 1980. Issues in the comparative measurement of political democracy. *American Sociological Review*, 45, 370–90.

Bollen, K.A. 1989. *Structural Equation with Latent Variables*. New York: Wiley.

Bollen, K.A. 1990. Political democracy: conceptual and measurement traps. *Studies in Contemporary International Development*, 25 (1), 7–24.

Bongaarts, J. 1978. A framework for analyzing the proximate determinants of fertility. *Population and Development Review*, 4 (1), 105–32.

Bonn International Center for Conversion (BICC). 2009. Migration and Displacement in Sub-Saharan Africa. Available at: www.reliefweb.int/rw/rwb.nsf.

Boon, B. and Tan, L. 2002. Impact of industrialization on acculturation of managers in the global marketplace. *Singapore Management Review*, 24 (1), 1–25.

Boserup, E. 1970. *Women's Role in Economic Development*. New York: St. Martin's.

Bowman, O.C. 2000. Peruvian female industrialists and the globalization project: deindustrialization and women's independence. *Gender and Society*, 14 (4), 540–59.

Bradley, K. and Ramirez, F.O. 1996. World polity and gender parity: women's share of higher education, 1965–1985. *Research in Sociology of Education and Socialization*, 11, 63–91.

Breen, N. 2002. Social discrimination and health: gender, race, and class in the United States, in *Engendering International Health: The Challenge of Equity*, edited by G. Sen, A. George, and P. Ostlin. Cambridge, MA: MIT Press, 223–55.

Brodie, J. 1996. Restructuring and the new citizenship, in *Rethinking Restructuring Gender and Change in Canada*, edited by I. Bakker. Toronto: University of Toronto Press, 126–40.

Burke, E. 1790. *Reflection on the Revolution in France*. Available at: http://www.constitution.org/eb/rev_fran.htm.

Caldwell, J.C. 1986. Routes to low mortality in poor countries. *Population and Development Review*, 12, 171–220.

Caldwell, J.C. 1992. Old and new factors in health transitions. *Health Transition Review*, 2, supplementary issue, 205–15.

Caldwell, J.C. 2001. Population health transition. *Bulletin of the World Health Organization,* 79 (2), 159–60.

Camacho, A.V., Castro, M.D. and Kaufman, R. 2006. Cultural aspects related to the health of Andean women in Latin America: a key issue for progress toward the attainment of the Millennium Development Goals. *International Journal of Gynecology and Obstetrics*, 94, 357–63.

Carlough, M. and McCall, M. 2005. Skilled birth attendance: what does it mean and how can it be measured? A clinical skills assessment of maternal and child health workers in Nepal. *International Journal of Gynecology and Obstetrics*, 89, 200–08.

Carmine, E.G. and Zeller, R.A. 1979. *Reliability and Validity Assessment*. Newbury Park, CA: Sage.

Castells, M. 1996. *The Rise of the Network Society*. Oxford, UK: Blackwell.

Castle, S., Traore, S. and Cisse, L. 2002. (Re) defining reproductive health with and for the community: an example of participatory research from Mali. *African Journal of Reproductive Health*, 6 (1), 20–31.

Castro, F.G. and Alarcon, E.H. 2002. Integrating cultural variables into drug abuse prevention and treatment with racial/ethnic minorities. *Journal of Drug Issues,* 32 (3), 783–810.

Center for Reproductive Law and Policy (CRLP). 2000. *Convention on the Elimination of All Forms of Discrimination against Women*. Available at: www.crlp.org/pub.fac_cedaw.html.

Center for Reproductive Rights. 2008. *The World's Abortion Laws*. Available at: www.reproductiverights.org.

Centers for Disease Control and Prevention (CDC). 2006a. *Reproductive Health Indicators*. Available at: http://www.cdc.gov/reproductivehealth/gisatlas/indicators.htm.

Centers for Disease Control and Prevention (CDC). 2006b. *Reproductive Health in Refugee Populations*. Available at: www.cdc.gov/reproductivehealth/refugee/index.htm.

Chafetz, J.S. 1984. *Sex and Advantage: A Comparative, Macro-Structural Theory of Sex Stratification*. Totowa, NJ: Rowman and Allanheld.

Chafetz, J.S. 1988. The gender division of labor and the reproduction of female disadvantage: toward an integrated theory. *Journal of Family Issues*, 9 (1), 108–31.

Chafetz, J.S. 1990. *Gender Equity: A Theory of Stability and Change*. Newbury Park, CA: Sage.

Chafetz, J.S. 1991. The gender division of labor and the reproduction of female disadvantage: toward an integrated theory, in *Gender, Family, and Economy: The Triple Overlap*, edited by R.L. Blumberg. Newbury Park, CA: Sage, 74–94.

Chafetz, J.S. 1997. Feminist theory and sociology: underutilized contributions for mainstream theory. *Annual Review of* Sociology, 23, 97–120.

Charles, M. 1992. Cross-national variations in occupational sex segregation. *American Sociological Review,* 57, 483–502.

Chatterjee, N. and Riley, N. 2001. Planning an Indian modernity: the gendered politics of fertility control. *Signs*, 26 (3), 812–45.

Chen, L.C., Evans, T, Anand, S., Boufford, J.I., Brown, H., Chowhury, M., Cueto, M., Dare, C., Dussault, G., Elzinga, G., Fee, E., Habte, D., Hanvoravongchai, P., Jacobs, M., Kurowski, C., Michael, S., Pablos-Mendez, A., Sewankambo, N., Salimano, G., Stilwell, B., Waal, A. and Wibulpolpraset, S. 2004. Human resources for health: overcoming the crisis. *The Lancet*, 364 (27), 1984–90.

Chen, S. and Ravallion, M. 2008. The developing world is poorer than we thought, but no less successful in the fight against poverty. *Policy Research Paper 4703*. Washington, DC: World Bank. Available at: www.doin.com/p–6223993.html.

Cincotta, R.P. and Crane, B.B. 2001. The Mexico City policy and U.S. family planning assistance. *Science*, 294, 525–6.

Cingranelli, D.L. and Richards, D.L. 2008. *CIRI Human Rights Data Project*. Available at: http://ciri.binghamton.edu/documentation.asp.

Claeson, M., Bos, E.R., Mawji, T. and Pathmanathan, I. 2000. Reducing child mortality in India in the new millennium. *Bulletin of the World Health Organization,* 78 (1), 1192–202.

Clark, R. 1991. Contrasting perspectives on women's access to prestigious occupations: a cross-national investigation. *Social Science Quarterly,* 72, 20–32.

Clark, R., Ramsbey, T.W. and Adler, E.S. 1991. Culture, gender, and labor force participation: a cross-national study. *Gender and Society,* 5, 47–66.

Coale, A.J. 1973. The demographic transition. *International Population Conference*, 1, 53–72.

Coleman, J. 1971. The development syndrome: differentiation – equality – capacity, in *Crises and Sequences in Political Development*, edited by L. Binder, J.S. Coleman, J. LaPalombara, L.W. Pye, S. Verba and M. Weiner. Princeton, NJ: Princeton University Press, 73–100.

Collins, R. 1986. *Weberian Sociological Theory*. New York: Cambridge University Press.

Collins, R., Chafetz, J.S., Blumberg, R.L., Coltrane, S. and Turner, J. 1993. Toward an integrated theory of gender stratification. *Sociological Perspectives*, 36, 185–216.

Collins, R. and Makowsky, M. 1993. *The Discovery of Society* (5th ed). New York: McGraw-Hill.

Commission on Social Determinants of Health (CSDH), World Health Organization (WHO). 2008. *Challenges to Implementing the "Social Determinants for Health Equity" (SDHE) Agenda in Countries*. Available at: www.who.int/social_determinants/media/sche_report_with_annexes_june_meeting_2008.pdf.

Comte, A. 1851. *System of Positive Philosophy*. New York: Burt Franklin.

Condorcet, M. 1790. On giving women the right of citizenship, in *Condorcet, Foundations of Social Choice and Political Theory*, edited and translated by I. McLean and F. Hewitt (1994). Aldershot, UK: Edward Elgar Publishing, 333–39.

Cook, R.J. 1993. International human rights and women's reproductive health. *Studies in Family Planning,* 24, 73–86.

Cook, R.J. 1995. Gender, health, and human rights. *Health and Human Rights*, 1 (4), 350–66.

Cook, R.J. and Bernard, D. 2003. Human rights dynamics of abortion law reform. *Human Rights Quarterly*, 25 (1), 1–59.

Cook, T.D. and Campbell, D.T. 1979. *Quasi-experimentation: Design and Analysis Issues for Field Settings.* Skokie: Rand McNally.

Cooley, C.H. 1902 (1964). *Human Nature and Social Order.* New York: Scribner's.

Cooley, C.H. 1909. *Social Organization.* New York: Schocken Book.

Cornia, G.A., Rosignoli, S. and Tiberti, L. 2007. Globalization and health: pathways of transmission and evidence of impact. *Globalization Knowledge Network Research Papers, WHO Commission on Social Determinants of Health.* Available at: www.who.int/social_determinants/resources.gkn_cornia_al.pdf.

Correa, S. and Petchesky, R. 1994. Reproductive and sexual rights: a feminist perspective, in *Population Policies Reconsidered: Health, Empowerment, and Rights*, edited by G. Sen, A. Germain, and L.C. Chen. Boston: Harvard University Press, 107–23.

Cotter, D.A., Hermsen, J.G., Joan, G., Ovadia, S. and Venneman, R. 2001. The glass ceiling effect. *Social Forces*, 80 (2), 655–82.

Cottingham, J., Hilbert, M.A., Colombini, M. and Kismodi, E. 2002. Gender and reproductive rights in reproductive health. *Annual Technical Report* 2002.

Cottingham, J. and Myntti, C. 2002. Reproductive health: conceptual mapping and evidence, in *Engendering International Health: The Challenge of Equity*, edited by G. Sen, A. George, and P. Ostlin. Cambridge, MS: MIS Press, 83–109.

Crane, B.B. and Dusenberry, J. 2004. Power and politics in international funding for reproductive health: the US Global Gag Rule. *Reproductive Health Matters*, 12 (24): 128–37.

Curtis, S. 2004. *Health and Inequality: Geographical Perspectives*, Thousand Oaks, CA: Sage.

Dahrendorf, R. 1989. *The Modern Social Conflict: An Essay on the Politics of Liberty.* Berkley, CA: University of California Press.

Davidson, S. and Lush, L. 1995. What Is Reproductive Care? *Refugee Participation Network*, 20, 4–8.

Davis, K. and Blake, J. 1956. Social structural and fertility: an analytic framework. *Economics Development and Cultural Change*, 4 (4), 211–35.

de Beauvoir, S. 1949. *The Second Sex* (translated by H.M. Parshley 1952). New York: Vintage Books.

de Gouges, O. 1791. The declaration of the rights of women, in *The French Revolution and Human Rights: A Brief Documentary History*, edited and translated by L. Hunt (1996). Boston/New York: St. Martin's, 124–29. Also available at www.fordham.edu/hslsall/mod/degorge.html.

Demakakos, P., Nazroo, J., Breeze, E. and Marmot, M. 2008. Socioeconomic status and health: the role of subjective social status. *Social Science and Medicine*, 67, 330–40.

Diamond, L., Linz, J. and Lipset, S.M. (eds). 1988–9. *Democracy in Developing Countries* (3 volumes). Boulder, CO: Lynne Rienner.

Diamond, L., Linz, J. and Lipset, S.M. 1990. *Politics in Developing Countries: Comparing Experiences with Democracy*. Boulder, CO: Lynne Rienner.

Diamond, L. and Marks, G. 1992. Seymour Martin Lipset and the study of democracy, in *Reexamining Democracy: Essays in Honor of Seymour Martin Lipset*, edited by G. Marks and L. Diamond. Thousand Oaks, CA: Sage.

Dijkstra, G.A. and Hanmer, L.C. 2000. Measuring socio-economic gender inequality: toward an alternative to the UNDP gender-related development index. *Feminist Economics*, 6 (2), 41–75.

Dixon-Mueller, R. 1993. *Population Policy and Women's Rights*. Westport, CT: Praeger.

Dixon-Mueller, R. 1998. *Female Empowerment and Demographic Process: Moving Beyond Cairo*. Policy and Research Papers No. 13. Paris: IUSSP.

Dixon-Mueller, R. and Germain, A. 2006. Fertility regulation and reproductive health in the Millennium development: the search for a perfect indicator? *American Journal of Public Health*, 97 (1), 45–51.

Dixon-Mueller, R. and Wasserheit, J. 1991. *The Culture of Silence: Reproductive Tract Infections among Women in the Third World*. New York: International Women's Health Coalition.

Dunn, D., Almquist, E.M. and Chafetz, J.S. 1993. Macrostructural perspectives on gender inequality, in *Theory on Gender / Feminism on Theory*, edited by P. England. New York: Aldine de Gruyter, 69–90.

Durkheim, E. 1893/1964. *The Division of Labor in Society* (translated by G. Simpson). Glencoe: The Free Press.

Durkheim, E. 1897/1957. *Suicide: A Study in Sociology*, Glencoe: The Free Press.

Dyson, T. and Moore, M. 1983. On kinship structure, female autonomy, and demographic behavior in India. *Population and Development Review*, 9 (1), 35–60.

Easley, C.E., Marks, S.P. and Morgan, R. 2001. The challenge and place of international human rights in public health. *American Journal of Public Health*, 91 (12), 1922–25.

Ebaugh, H.R. and Chafetz, J.S. 1999. Agents for cultural reproduction and structural change: the ironic role of women in immigrant religious institutions. *Social Forces*, 78 (2), 585–613.

Ehrlich, P.R. 1968. *The Population Bomb*, Cutchogue, NY: Ballantine Books.

Ehrlich, P.R. and Ehrlich, A.H. 1972. *Population, Resources, Environment: Issues in Human Ecology* (2nd ed.). San Francisco, CA: W.H. Freeman and Company.

Ellaway, A. and Mackintye, S. 1996. Does where you live predict health related behaviors? A case study in Glagow. *Health Bull*, 54, 443–46.

Elliot, P. and Wartenberg, D. 2004. Spatial epidemiology: current approaches and future challenge. *Environmental Health Perspectives*, 112 (9), 998–1006.

England, P. 2000. Conceptualizing women's empowerment in countries of the north, in *Women's Empowerment and Demographic Processes*, edited by H. Presser and G. Sen. New York: Oxford University Press.

Entwisle, B., Gail, E., Henderson, S.E., Short, Bouma, J. and Zhai, F.Y. 1995. Gender and family business in rural China. *American Sociological Review*, 60, 36–57.

Esscher, A.O. 2004. *Reproductive Health in Humanitarian Assistance*. Available at: www.kbh.uu.se/imch/phha/phha.html.

Estes, R.J. 1984. *The Social Progress of Nations*. New York: Praeger.

Estes, R.J. 2007. Asia and the new century: challenges and opportunities. *Social Indicators Research*, 82, 375–410.

FAFIA-AFAI. 2007. *Social Watch Gender Equity Index: Inequality Persists*. Available at: www.fafia-afai.org/en/social_watch_gender_equity_index_inequality_persists.

Fathalla, M.F. 1992. Reductive health: a global overview. *Human Development*, 29, 35–42.

Fathalla, M.F. 1993. Contraception and women's health. *British Medical Bulletin*, 49, 245–51.

Feitshans, I.L. 1998. Is there a human right to reproductive health? *Texas Journal of Women and Law*, 8 (1), 93–133.

Ferree, M.M. 1990. Beyond separate spheres: feminism and family research. *Journal of Marriage and the Family*, 52, 866–84.

Ferree, M.M. and Hall, E.J. 1996. Rethinking stratification from a feminist perspective: gender, race, and class in mainstream textbooks. *American Sociological Review*, 61 (6), 929–50.

Filmer, R. 1680 (printed). *Patriarcha or the Natural Power of Kings*. Available at: www.constitution.org/eng/patriarcha.htm.

Fitzpatrick, K.M. and LaGory, M. 2003. Placing health in an urban sociology: cities as mosaics of risk and protection. *City and Society*, 2, 33.

Folbre, N. 1983. Of patriarchy born: the political economy of fertility decisions. *Feminist Studies*, l9, 261–84.

Forsythe, N., Korzeniewicz, R.P. and Durrant, V. 2000. Gender inequalities and economic growth: a longitudinal evaluation. *Economic Development and Cultural Change*, 48 (3), 573–617.

Fossedal, G.A. 1989. *The Democratic Imperative: Exporting the American Revolution*. New York: Basic Books.

Fox-Harding, L. 1996. *Family, State, and Social Policy*. Basingstoke: Macmillan.

Fox-Piven, F. 1990. Ideology and the state: women, power and the welfare state, in *Women, the State and the Welfare*, edited by L. Gorgon. Madison, WI: University of Wisconsin Press.

Frank, A.G. 1967. *Capitalism and Underdevelopment in Latin America*. New York and London: Monthly Review Press.

Freedom House. 2000. *A Survey of Global Political Change in the 20th Century*. Available at: www.freedomhouse.org/reports/country.html.

Freedom House. 2007. *Freedom in the World.* Available at: www.freedomhouse.org.

Freeman, L.P. and Isaacs, S.L. 1993. Human rights and reproductive choice. *Studies in Family Planning*, 24 (1), 18–30.

Friedan, B. 1963. *The Feminine Mystique*. New York: W.W. Norton and Company, Inc.

García-Moreno, C. and Claro, A. 1994. Challenges from the women's health movement: women's rights versus population control. Available at: http://www.hsph.harvard.edu/rt21/globalism/CLARO.html.

Gastil, R.D. 1988. *Freedom in the World: Political Rights and Civil Liberties, 1987–1988*. New York: Freedom House.

Germain, A., Nowrojee, S. and Hnin, P. 1994. Setting a new agenda: sexual and reproductive health and rights, in *Population Policies Reconsidered: Health, Empowerment, and Rights*, edited by G. Sen, A. German and L.C. Chen. Boston: Harvard University Press, 27–46.

Germain, A. and Dixon-Mueller, R. 2005. Reproductive health and the MDGs: is the glass half full or half empty? *Studies in Family Planning*, 36 (2), 137–40.

Ghoshal, B. 2004. Democratic transition and political development in post-Soeharto Indonesia. *Contemporary Southeast Asia*, 26 (3), 506–29.

Gibson, M. 2007. *Culture and Power: A History of Culture Studies*. Sydney: University of New South Wale Press.

Gilman, C.P. 1898. *Women and Economics: A Study of the Economic Relation between Men and Women as a Factor in Social Evolution*. Boston: Small Maynard and Co.

Glasier, A., Gulmezoglu, A.M., Schmid, G.P., Moreno, C.G., Look, P.F.V. 2006. Sexual and productive health: a matter of life and death. *The Lancet*, 368 (9547), 1595–607.

Goesling, B. and Firebaugh, G. 2004. The trend in international health inequality. *Population and Development Review*, 30 (1): 131–46.

Goldberg, C.A. 2001. Social citizenship and a reconstructed Tocqueville. *American Sociological Review*, 66 (2), 289–315.

Gordon, L. 1974. The politics of population: birth control and the eugenics movement. *Radical America*, 8 (4), 61–97.

Gostin, L. 2000. *Public Health Law: Power, Duty, Restraint*. New York: University of California Press and the Milbank Memorial Fund.

Gottlieb, P. and Lindmark, G. 2002. WHO indicators for evaluation of maternal health care services. Applicability in least developed countries: a case study from Eritrea. *African Journal of Reproductive Health*, 6 (2), 13–22.

Gould, M.I. and Jones, K. 1996. Analyzing perceived limiting long-term illness using U.K. census Microdata. *Social Science and Medicine*, 42 (6), 867–69.

Greenhalgh, S. 1990. Toward a political economy of fertility: anthropological contributions. *Population and Development Review*, 16 (1), 85–106.

Greissimer, T.O. 1954. *The Population Bomb*. New York: IPPF.

Gribble, J. and Haffey, J. 2008. Reproductive health in sub-Saharan Africa. *BRIDGE* (Bringing Information to Decisionmakers for Global Effectiveness), Population Reference Bureau, 1–4. Available at: www.prb.org/pdf08/reproductive health_subsaharanafrica.pdf.

Hagoplan, F. 2000. Political development, revisited. *Comparative Political Studies*, 33 (6/7), 880–911.

Hakim, C. 1998. Developing a sociology for the twenty-first century: preference theory. *British Journal of Sociology,* 49, 137–43.

Hanefeld, J., Spicer, N., Brugha, R. and Walt, G. 2007. *How have Global Health Initiatives Impacted on Health Equity? What Strategies can be Put in Place to Enhance their Positive Impact and Mitigate against Negative Impacts*? Available at: www.who.int/social_determinants/resources/csch_media/global_health_initiatives_2007_en.pdf.

Haney, L.A. 2000. Feminist state theory: applications to jurisprudence, criminology, and the welfare state. *Annual Review of Sociology*, 26, 641–66.

Hansluwka, H. 1985. Measuring the health of populations: indicators and interpretations. *Social Science and Medicine*, 20 (12), 1207–224.

Hardin, G. 1968. The tragedy of the commons. *Science*, 162 (3859), 1243–248.

Harris, C. and Smyth, I. 2001. The reproductive health of refugees: lessons beyond ICPD. *Gender and Development*, 9 (2), 10–21.

Hartmann, B. 1987. *Reproductive Rights and Wrongs*. New York: Harper and Row.

Harvey, D. 2000. *Spaces of Hope*. Berkeley, CA: University of California Press.

Hellsten, S.K. 2000. Women's rights and reproductive care in a global perspective. *Journal of Social Philosophy*, 31 (4), 382–90.

Hess, B. and Ferree, M.M. (eds) 1987. *Analyzing Gender: A Handbook of Social Science Research*. Newbury Park, CA: Sage.

Higer, A.J. 1995. U.S. population policy and feminism: a working relationship? *Political Environments #2*. Available at: http://www.cwpe.org/issues/population_html/higer.html.

Hobbes, T. 1660. *The Leviathan*. Available at: http://etext.library.adelaide.edu.au/h/h681/h681.html.

Hobson, B. 1994. Solo mothers, social policy regimes and the logics of gender, in *Gendering Welfare States*, edited by D. Sainsbury. London: Sage, 170–87.

Hodgson, D. and Watkins, S.C. 1997. Feminists and neo-Malthusians: past and present alliances. *Population and Development Review*, 23 (3), 469–524.

Homer-Dixon, T.F. 1991. On the threshold: environmental changes as causes of acute conflict. *Trudeau Centre for Peace and Conflict Studies, University of Toronto International Security*, 16 (2), 76–116.

Homer-Dixon, T.F. 2000. *The Ingenuity Gap: Facing the Economic, Environmental, and Other Challenges of an Increasingly Complex and Unpredictable World.* New York: Knopf Publishing Group.

Howard, R.E. 1995. Women's rights and right to development, in *Women's Rights and Human Rights*, edited by J. Peters and A. Wolper. New York: Routledge.

Hume, D. 1739–40. *A Treatise of Human Nature*. Available at: http://etext.lib.adelaide.edu.au/h/hume/david/h92t/index/html.

Huntington, E. 2001. *Civilization and Climate*. Portland, OR: University Press of Pacific.

Hutt, C. 1976. *Males and Females*. Harmondsworth: Penguim Education.

Hwang, A.C. and Stewart, F.H. 2004. Family planning in balance. *American Journal of Public Health*, 94 (1), 15–8.

Hyde, J., Fennema, E. and Laman, S.J. 1990. Gender differences in mathematics performance: a meta-analysis. *Psychological Bulletin*, 107, 139–50.

Inglehart, R. and Norris, P. 2003. *Rising Tide: Gender Equality and Cultural Change around the World*. Cambridge: Cambridge University Press.

International Federation of Gynecology and Obstetrics (FIGO). 2006. *World Report on Women's Health*. Available at: www.figo.org/publications/world.

International Labor Organization (ILO). 1951. *Convention Concerning Equal Remuneration for Men and Women Workers for Work of Equal Value*. Available at: http://www.ilo/org.

International Labor Organization (ILO). 1958. *Recommendation Concerning Discrimination in Respect of Employment and Occupation*. Available at: http://www.ilo.org.

International Planned Parenthood Federation (IPPF). 2000a. *IPPF Charter on Sexual and Reproductive Rights*. London: Banson.

International Planned Parenthood Foundation (IPPF). 2000b. *Sexual and Reproductive Health Indicator Development*. Available at: www.ippfwhr.org.

International Planned Parenthood Foundation (IPPF). 2002. Men as partners for gender equity. *Report of the IPPF International-Regional Workshop Group Meeting*. New York: IPPF.

Jacobson, J.L. 2000. Transforming family planning programs: towards a framework for advancing the reproductive rights agenda. *Reproductive Health Matters*, 8 (15), 21–32.

Jameson, K.P. 1996. Data and social science rhetoric: policy and instruction. *IASSIST Quarterly*, 20 (1), 18–24.

Jamieson, D.J., Meikle, S.F., Hills, S.D., Mtsuko, D., Mawji, S. and Duerr, A. 2000. An evaluation of poor pregnancy outcome among Burundian refugees in Tanzania. *Journal of the American Medical Association* (JAMA), 283 (3), 397–402.

Jaquette, J.S. and Wolchik, S.L. (eds). 1998. *Women and Democracy: Latin America and Central and Eastern Europe*. Baltimore: Johns Hopkins University Press.

Jejeebhoy, S.J. 2000. Women's autonomy in rural India: its dimensions, determinants, and the influence of context, in *Women's Empowerment and Demographic Processes: Moving Beyond Cairo*, edited by H. Presser and G. Sen. New York: Oxford University Press.

Jensen, J. 1995. Extending the boundaries of citizenship: women's movements in Western Europe, in *The Challenge of Local Feminisms: Women's Movements in Global Perspectives,* edited by A. Basu. Boulder, CO: Westview.

Joreskog, K.G. and Sorbom, D. 1989. *LISREL 7: A Guide to the Program and Applications* (2nd ed.). Chicago: SPSS Inc.

Kabeer, N. 1994. *Reversed Realities: Gender Hierarchies in Development Thought*. London: Verso.

Kahn, J., Johann, S., Arnason, P., Elsenstadt, S.N. and Englund, H. 2001. Anthropology and modernity. *Current Anthropology*, 42 (5), 651–80.

Kandal, T.R. 1988. *The Women Question in Classical Sociological Theory*. Miami, FL: Florida International University Press.

Kant, I. 1788. *The Critique of Practical Reason* (translated by W.S. Pluhar 1956). New York: Liberal Arts Press.

Keleher, H. and Franklin, L.J. 2008. Changing gendered norms about girls at the level of household and community: a review of the evidence. *Global Public Health* 3(S1), 42–57.

Kerr, C.l., Dunlop, J.T., Harbison, F.H. and Myers, C.A. 2001. Industrialism and industrial man, in *Social Stratification: Class, Race, and Gender,* edited by D.B. Grusky. Boulder, CO: Westview, 793–804.

Kerr, J. and Sweetman, C. 2003. Editorial. *Gender and Development*, 11 (1), 3–12.

Khattab, H. 1992. *Silent Endurance: the Social Conditions of Women's Reproductive Health*. Amman: UNCIEF.

Kickbusch, I. 2004. The end of public health as we know it: constructing global health in the 21st century. *Hugh R. Leavell Lecture Series, World Federation of Public Health Association (WFPHA) 10th International Congress on Public Health*. Available at: http://sdnhq.undp.org/gpgn/r-health.php.

Kishor, S. 2000. Empowerment of women in Egypt and links to the survival and health of their infants, in *Women's Empowerment and Demographic Processes: Moving beyond Cairo*, edited by H. Presser and G. Sen. New York: Oxford University Press.

Klitsch, M. 1999. The bumpy road from Cairo to now and beyond. *International Family Planning Perspectives,* 25 (4), 196–206.

Krause, S.K., Jones, R.K. and Purdin, S. 2000. Programmatic responses to refugees' reproductive health needs *International Family Planning Perspectives,* 26 (4), 181–7.

Kritz, M.M., Makinwa-Adebusoye, P. and Gurak, D.T. 2000. The role of gender context in shaping reproductive behavior in Nigeria, in *Women's Empowerment and Demographic Processes*, edited by H. Presser and G. Sen. New York: Oxford University Press.

Lamas, M. 2001. Standing fast in Mexico: protecting women's rights in a hostile climate. *NACLA Report on the Americas*, 34 (5), 36–40.

Lane, S.D. 1994. From population control to reproductive health: an emerging policy agenda. *Social Science and Medicine*, 39, 1303–314.

Langermann, P.M. and Niebrugge-Brantley, J. 1992. Contemporary feminist theory, in *Sociological Theory* (3rd ed.), edited by G. Ritzer. New York: McGraw-Hill, 447–96.

Lavee, Y. 1988. Linear structural relationships (LISREL) in family research. *Journal of Marriage and the Family*, 50 (4), 937–48.

Lerner, D. 1968. *The Passing of Traditional Society: Modernizing the Middle East*. New York: The Free Press.

Lewis, G. 2000. Expanding the social policy imaginary, in *Rethinking Social Policy*, edited by G. Lewis, S. Gewirtz, and J. Clarke. Thousand Oaks, CA: Sage, 1–21.

Lewis, J. 2000. Gender and welfare regimes in rethinking social policy, in *Rethinking Social Policy*, edited by G. Lewis, S. Gewirtz, and J. Clarke. Thousand Oaks, CA: Sage, 27–51.

Lipset, S.M. 1959. Some social requisites of democracy: economic development and political legitimacy. *The American Political Science Review,* 53 (1), 69–105.

Lipset, S.M. 1960. *Political Man: The Social Bases of Politics*. New York: Doubleday.

Lipset, S.M. 1983. *Political Man: The Social Bases of Politics* (expanded and updated edition). London: Heinemann.

Lister, R. 2000. Gender and the analysis of social policy, in *Rethinking Social Policy,* edited by G. Lewis, S. Gewirtz, and J. Clarke. Thousand Oaks, CA: Sage, 22–36.

Locke, J. 1690. *Two Treatises of Government*. Available at: http://etext.lib.virginia.edu/toc/modeng/public/LocTre2.html.

Luciak, I.A. 1999. Gender equality in the Salvadoran transition. *Latin American Perspectives,* 26 (2), 43–67.

Luke, T.W. 1990. *Social Theory and Modernity*. Newbury Park, CA: Sage.

Lynn, R. 1994. Sex differences in intelligence and brain size: a paradox resolved. *Personality and Individual Differences*, 17, 257–71.

Macintyre, S. 1997. The Black report and beyond: what are the issues? *Social Science and Medicine*, 44 (6), 723–45.

Malhotra, A. and Mehra, R. 1999. *Fulfilling the Cairo Commitment: Enhancing Women's Economic and Social Options for Better Reproductive Health*. Washington, D.C.: International Center for Research on Women.

Malhotra, A., Schuler, S.R. and Boender, C. 2002. Measuring women's empowerment as a variable in international development. Commissioned Paper of the Gender and Development Group of the World Bank. Available at: http://www.icrw.org/docs/measuringempowerment_workingpaper_802.doc.

Malthus, T.R. 1798. *An Essay on the Principle of Population*. Available at: http://socserv2.socsci.mcmaster.ca/~econ/ugcm/3113/malthus/popu.txt.

Mann, J. 1996. Human rights and aids: the future of the pandemic. *The John Marshall Law Review,* 30, 195–206.

Mann, J. 1997. Medicine and public health, ethics and human rights. *Hastings Center Report,* 27, 6–13.

Mann, J., Gostin, L., Gruskin, S., Brennan, T., Lazzarini, Z. and Fineberg, H. 1999. Health and human rights, in *Health and Human Rights,* edited by J.M. Mann, S. Gruskin, M.A. Grodin, and G.J. Annas. New York: Routledge, 7–20.

Margolis, L.H., Gay, K. and Humphrey, A.D. 1998. The role of state maternal and child health programs in the issue of newborn discharge. *Maternal and Child Health Journal*, 2 (1), 45–54.

Marks, S.P. 2001a. The new partnership of health and human rights. *Human Rights Dialogue Series*, 2 (6), 21–22.

Marks, S.P. 2001b. Jonathan Mann's legacy to the 21st century: the human rights imperative for public health. *The Journal of Law, Medicine and Ethics*, 29 (2), 131–8.

Marmalakis, M. 1996. Misuse and use of national accounts as a welfare indicator: selected analytical and measurement issues. *Review of Income and Wealth*, 42 (3), 293–320.

Marshall, T.H. 1964. *Class, Citizenship, and Social Development: Essays by Thomas H. Marshall*. Garden City, NY: Anchor Books.

Maruyama, G.M. 1997. *Basics of Structural Equation Modeling*. Thousand Oaks, CA: Sage.

Marx, K. and Engels, F. 1848. *The Communist Manifesto*. New York: Barron's Educational Series.

Mason, K.O. 1984. *The Status of Women: A Review of its Relationship in Mortality and Fertility*. New York: The Rockefeller Foundation.

Mason, K.O. 1986. The status of women: conceptual and methodological issues in demographic studies. *The Eastern Sociological Society*, 1 (2), 284–300.

Mason, K.O. 1993. The impact of women's position on demographic change during the course of development, in *Women's Position and Demographic Change*, edited by N. Federici, K.O. Mason, and S. Sogner. Oxford: Clarendon Press.

Mason, K.O. 1998. Wives' economic decision-making power in the family: five Asian countries, in *The Changing Family in Comparative Perspective: Asia and the United States*, edited by K.O. Mason. Honolulu: East-West Center,105–33.

Mason, K.O. and Smith, H.L. 2003. *Women's Empowerment and Social Context: Results from Five Asian Countries*. Available at: http://swaf.pop.upenn.edu/publicationspage.html.

Mass, B. 1972. *The Political Economy of Population Control in Latin America*. Toronto: Women's Press.

Matthew, R.A. 2000. Environment and security in an international context: critiquing a pilot study from NATO's committee on the challenges of modern society. *Environmental Change and Security Project Report*, 6, 95–103.

Matthews, S., Ribar, D. and Wilhelm, M. 1997. The effects of economic conditions and access to reproductive health services on state abortion rates and birthrates. *Family Planning Perspectives,* 29, (2), 52–60.

McDaniel, S.A. 1996. Toward a synthesis of feminist and demographic perspectives on fertility. *The Sociological Quarterly,* 37 (1), 83–104.

McDaniel, S.A. 2002. Women's changing relations to the state and citizenship: caring and intergenerational relations in globalizing western democracies. *The Canadian Review of Sociology and Anthropology,* 39 (2), 125–50.

McDonagh, J. 2002. *Renegotiating Rural Development in Ireland.* England: Ashagate Publishing.

McKee, M., Balabanova, D., Akingbade, K., Pomerleau, J., Stickley, A., Rose, R. and Haerpfer, C. 2006. Access to water in the countries of the former Soviet Union. *Public Health*, 120, 364–72.

McKeown, T. 1979. *The Role of Medicine: Dream, Mirage, or Nemesis*. New York: Tavistock.

McKeown, T. 1991. *The Origin of Human Diseases*. San Francisco, CA: Wiley-Blackwell.

McMichael, A., McKee, M., Skolnokov, V. and Valkonen, K. 2004. Mortality trends and setbacks: global convergence or divergence? *The Lancet*, 363 (9415): 1155–59.

Mead, G.H. 1934. *Mind, Self, and Society*. Chicago: University of Chicago Press.

Medel-Anonuevo, C. (ed.). 1995. *Women, Education and Empowerment*. Hamburg, Germany: UNESCO Institute for Education.

Merali, I. 2000. Advancing women's reproductive and sexual health rights: using the international human rights system. *Development in Practice*, 10 (5), 609–24.

Mills, W.C. 1961. *The Sociological Imagination*. New York: Grove Press.

Mommsen, W. 1974. *The Age of Bureaucracy: Perspectives on the Political Sociology of Max Weber*. New York: Harper and Row.

Monroe, P.A. 1996. *Left-brain Finances for Right-brain People: A Guide for the Creatively Inclined.* Naperville, IL: Sourcebooks.

Moore, H. 1956. *The Population* Bomb. New York: Hugh Moore Fund.

Moore, W.E. 1965. *The Impact of Industry*. Englewood, CA: Prentice-Hall.

Morgan, V. 2001. Introduction to the UNDP's gender empowerment measure and the gender development index, in UNDP *Measuring Women's Empowerment*, 1–4. Available at: http://www.gweb.kvinnoforum.se/papers/measuringwomensempowerment2001.pdf.

Morrisson, C. and Jutting, J. 2005. Women's discrimination in developing countries: a new data set for better policies. *World Development*, 33 (7), 1065–81.

Mosley, W.H. and Chen, L.C. (eds). 1984. *Child Survival: Strategies for Research Supplement to Population and Development Review 10*. New York: The Population Council.

Moussa, G. 2008. Gender aspects of human security. *International Social Science Journal*, 59 (193), 81–100.

NcFarlane, D.R. and Meier, K. J. 2001. *The Politics of Fertility Control.* New York: Chatham House Publishers.

Nelson, H.L. 2000. Feminist bioethics: where we've been, where we're going. *Metaphilosophy*, 31 (5), 492–508.

Nelson, J. 1987. *Social Origins of Dictatorship and Democracy: Lord and Peasant in the Making of the Modern World*. Boston: Beacon.

Nordhaus, W. 2000. New directions in national economic accounting. *American Economic Review*, 90 (2), 259–63.

Nordhaus, W. and Tobin, J. 1971. Is growth obsolete? *Cowles Foundation Discussion Paper No. 319*. New York: National Bureau of Economic Research. Available at: http://cowles.econ.yale.edu/P/cp/p03b/p0398ab.pdf.

Norris, P. 1987. *Politics and Sexual Equality*. London: Wheatsheaf.

Notestein, F.W. 1950. The population of the world in the year 2000. *American Statistical Association Journal*, 45, 335–45.

O'Donnell, G.A. and Schmitter, P.C. 1986. *Transitions from Authoritarian Rule: Tentative Conclusions about Uncertain Democracies*. Baltimore and London: Johns Hopkins University Press.

Obermeyer, C.M. 1999. The cultural context of reproductive health: implications for monitoring the Cairo agenda. *International Family Planning Perspectives*, 25, 50–55.

Omran, A.R. 1971. The epidemiological transition: a theory of the epidemiology of population change. *The Milbank Memorial Fund Quarterly,* 49 (4), 509–38.

Omran, A.R. 1982. Epidemiological transition, in *International Encyclopedia of Population*, Volume 1, edited by J.A. Ross. New York: The Free Press.

Orloff, A.S. 1993. Gender and the social rights of citizenship: the comparative analysis of gender relations and welfare states. *American Sociological Review*, 58, 303–28.

Osborn, F.H. 1960. *This Crowded World*. New York: Public Affairs Committee.

Orubuloye, I.O., Oguntimehin, E. and Sadique, T. 1997. Women's role in reproductive health decision making and vulnerability to STD and HIV/AIDS in Ekiti, Nigeria. *Health Transition Review,* 7, 329–36.

Östlin, P. 2004. *Priorities for Research to Take forward the Health Equity Policy Agenda: Report from the WHO Take Force on Health System Research Priorities for Equity in Health*. Available at: www.who.int/rpc/meetings/en/Task_Force%20Report_Nov_Final[2].pdf.

Östlin, P., Schrecker, T. and Sadana, R. 2009. Priorities for research on equity and health: implications for global and national priority setting and the role of WHO to take the health equity research agenda forward. *Discussion Paper*. Geneva: World Health Organization.

Pachauri, S. 1999. *Implementing a Reproductive Health Agenda in India: The Beginning*. New Delhi: Population Council.

Pappa, G., Green S., Hadden, W. and Fisher, G. 1993. The increasing disparity in mortality between socioeconomic groups in the United States. *New England Journal of Medicine*, 329, 103–09.

Parker, R. 2001. Sexuality, culture, and power in HIV/AIDS research. *Annual Review of Anthropology,* 30, 163–79.

Parker, R. 2002. The global HIV/AIDS pandemic, structural inequalities and the politics of international health. *American Journal of Public Health,* 92 (3), 343–46.

Parsons, T. 1951. *The Social System*. New York: The Free Press.

Pearce, T.O. 2001. Human rights in sociology: some observations from Africa. *Social Problems*, 48 (1), 48–56.

Pearl, J. 2000. *Causality: Models, Reasoning, and Inference*, New York: Cambridge University Press.

Pedersen, J. 1987. Plantation women and children: wage labor, adoption, and fertility in the Seychelles. *Ethnology*, 26 (1), 51–61.

Penna, D.R. and Campbell, P.J. 1998. Human rights and culture: beyond university and relativism. *Third World Quarterly*, 19 (1), 7–27.

Petcheky, R.P. 1990. *Abortion and Women's Choice: The State, Sexuality, and Reproductive Freedom*. Boston, MA: Northeastern University Press.

Petchesky, R.P. 2000. Human rights, reproductive and sexual health and economic justice: why they are indivisible. *Reproductive Health Matters*, 8 (15), 1–9.

Peterson, V.P. 2003. *A Critical Rewriting of Global Political Economy: Integrating Reproductive, Productive and Virtual Economies*. London: Routledge/RIPE Series in Global Political Economy.

Phillips, A. 1991. *Engendering Democracy*. University Park, PA: Pennsylvania University Press.

Pickett, J.C., Reilly, D.P. and McIntyre, R.M. 2005. How to select most efficient OLS model for time series data. *The Journal of Business Forecasting*, Spring, 11–5.

Pillai, V.K. and Wang, G.Z. 1999. *Women's Reproductive Rights in Developing Countries*. Aldershot: Ashgate Publishing.

Pitanguy, J. 2002. Bridging the local and the global: feminism in Brazil and the international human rights agenda. *Social Research*, 69 (3), 805–20.

Poe, S.C., Tate, N. and Keith, L.C. 1999. Repression of the human right to personal integrity revisited: a global cross-national study covering the years 1976–1993. *International Studies Quarterly,* 43, 291–313.

Population Action International (PAI). 2001. *World of Difference: Sexual and Reproductive Health and Risks*. Available at: www.populationaction.org/resources/publications/worldofdifference.

Population Action International (PAI). 2009. *The Global Gag Rule Timeline Update*. Available at: www.populationaction.org/issues/U.S._Policies_and_funding/global_gag_rule.shtml.

Population Reference Bureau (PRB). 2002. *The World's Youth*. Available at: http://www.prb.org.

Population Resources Center (PRC). 2004. *World Population Trends*. Available at: http://www.prcdc.org.

Pratto, F., Stallworth, L.M., Sidanius, J. and Siers, B. 1997. The gender gap in occupational role attainment: a social dominance approach. *Journal of Personality and Social Psychology*, 72 (1), 37–53.

Presser, H. 1997. Demography, feminism, and the science – policy nexus. *Population and Development Review*, 23 (2), 295–331.

Qadeer, I. 1998. Reproductive health: a public health perspective. *Economic and Political Weekly,* 33 (41), 2675–84.

Ramirez, F.O., Soysal, Y. and Shanahan, S. 1997. The changing logic of political citizenship: cross-national acquisition of women's suffrage rights, 1890 to 1990. *American Sociological Review*, 62, 735–45.

Rao, A. and Kelleher, D. 2003. Institution, organizations and gender equality in an ear of globalization. *Gender and Development*, 11 (1), 142–9.

Rawls, J.B. 1971. *A Theory of Justice*. Cambridge, MA: Belknag Press of Harvard University Press.

Riley, N.E. 1997. Gender, power, and population change. *Population Bulletin*, 52 (1), 2–48.

Roberts, I. 1997. Cause specific social class mortality differentials for child injury and poisoning in England and Wales. *Journal of Epidemiological and Community Health*, 51 (3), 334–5.

Roberts, M.J. and Reich, M.R. 2002. Ethical analysis in public health. *The Lancet*, 359, 1055–9.

Rose, G.E. 1994. *The Strategy of Preventive Medicine*. New York: Oxford University Press.

Rosenfield, A. and Maine, D. 1985. Maternal mortality – a neglected tragedy, Where is the M in the MCH? *The Lancet*, II, 83–5.

Rosenfield, A. and Schwartz, K. 2005. Improving the health of women in developing countries: the time is now. *Journal of Midwifery and Women's Health*, 50 (4), 272–4.

Rousseau, J.J. 1754. *A Discourse on the Origin and Basis of Inequality among Men*. Available at: http://un2sg4.unige.ch/athena/rousseau/jjr_ineg.html.

Rousseau, J.J. 1762. *The Social Contract*. Available at: http://etext.library.adelaide.edu.au/r/rousseau/jean_jacques/r864s.

Rudd, E.C. 2000. Reconceptualizing gender in postsocialist transformation. *Gender and Society*, 14 (4), 517–39.

Sadik, N. 2000. Reproductive health and gender equality in the 21st century: a new reality. *International Lecture Series on Population Issues*, 4–15.

Safilios-Rothschild, C. 1982. Female power, autonomy and demographic change in the third world, in *Women's Roles and Population Trends in the Third World*, edited by R. Anker, M. Buvinic, and N.H. Youssef. London: Billing and Sons Limited, 117–132.

Sadana, R. 2002. Definition and measurement of reproductive health. *Bulletin of the World Health Organization*, 80 (5), 407–9.

Sartori, G. 1987. *The Theory of Democracy Revisited.* Chatham, NJ: Chatham House Publishers.

Save the Children. 2002. *State of the World's Mothers 2002: Mothers and Children in War and Conflict*. Available at: www.savethechildren.org/publications/mothers/2002/sowm2002.pdf.

Save the Children. 2003. *State of the World's Mothers 2002: Protecting Women and Children in War and Conflict*. Available at: www.planetwire/sowm–2003/sowm_2003.pdf.

Save the Children. 2009. Save the Children Report 2009. Available at: www.savethechidren.org/ publications/mothers/2009/sowm2009.pdf

Save the Children Fund. 2006. *Children's Rights Guide*. Available at: www.savethechildren.org.uk.

Say, L., Souza, J.P. and Patterson, R.C. 2009. Maternal near miss – towards a standard tool for monitoring quality of maternal health care. *Best Practice and Research Clinical Obstetrics and Gynaecology*, 23, 287–96.

Schaefer, M. 1998. *Health of Population*. Available at: http://depts.washington.edu/hserv/research/phdefinitions.shtml.

Schild, V. 2000. Gender equality without social justice: women's rights in the neoliberal age. *NACLA Report on the Americas,* 34 (1), 25–8.

Schrecker, T., Labonte, R. and De Vogli, R. 2008. Globalization and health: the need for a global vision. *The Lancet*, 372 (8), 1670–76.

Schultz, T. Paul (ed.) 1997. Investment in Women's Human Capital. Chicago: University of Chicago Press.

Schwartz, D.M., Deligiannis, T. and Homer-Dixon, T.F. 2000. The environment and violent conflict: a response to Gleditsch's critique and some suggestions for future research. *Environmental Change and Security Project Report* 6, 77–94.

Scott, G., Campbell, J. and Brown, U. 2002. Child care, social inclusion and urban regeneration. *Critical Social Policy*, 22 (2), 226–40.

Seidman, G.W. 1999. Gendered citizenship: South Africa's democratic transition and the construction of a gendered state. *Gender and Society*, 13 (3), 287–307.

Sen, A.K. 1973. *On Economic Inequality*. New York: Oxford University Press.

Sen, A.K. 1999. *Development as Freedom*. New York: Random House.

Sen, G. 1994. Reproduction: the feminist challenge to social policy, in *Power and Decision: The Social Control of Reproduction*, edited by G. Sen and R. Snow. Boston, MA: Harvard University Press, 5–17.

Sen, G. and Batliwala, S. 1990. Empowering women for reproductive rights, in *Women's Empowerment and Demographic Processes*, edited by H. Presser and G. Sen. New York: Oxford University Press.

Sen, G., George, A. and Ostlin, P. (eds). 2002. *Engendering International Health: The Challenge of Equity*. Boston, MA: MIT Press.

Sen, G. and Grown, C. 1987. *Development, Crises, and Alternative Visions: Third World Women's Perspectives*. New York: Monthly Review Press.

Shouls, S., Congdon, P. and Curtis, S. 1996. Modeling inequality in long term illness in UK: combating individual and area characteristics. *Journal of Epidemiology and Community Health*, 50, 366–77.

Sims, J. and Butter M.E. 2000. Gender equity and environmental health. *Harvard Center for Population and Development Studies Working Paper Series* June 2000, 1–24.

Sims J. and Butter M.E. 2002. Health and environment: moving beyond conventional paradigm, in *Engendering International Health: The Challenge of Equity*, edited by G. Sen, A. George, and P. Ostlin. Cambridge, MA: MIT Press, 195–220.

Sjoberg, G. and Vaughan, T.R. 1993. The ethical foundations of sociology and the necessity for human rights alternatives, in *A Critique of Contemporary American Sociology*, edited by T.R. Vaughan, G. Sjorberg, and L.T. Reynold. New York: Dix Hills, 114–59.

Slogett, A. and Joshi, H. 1998. Indicators of deprivation in people and places: longitudinal perspectives. *Environment and Planning*, 30, 1055–76.

Smith, J. and Ingham, L.H. 2005. Mothers' milk and measures of economic output. *Feminist Economics*, 11 (1), 41–62.

Smith, L.C., Ramarkrishnan, U., Ndiaye, A., Haddad, L. and Martorell, R. 2003. *The Importance of Women's Status for Child Nutrition in Developing Countries*. (Research Report 131). Available at: www.ifpri.org/pubs/abstract/abstr131.htm.

Sorensen, G. 1993. *Democracy and Democratization: Processes and Prospects in a Changing World.* Boulder, CO: Westview Press.

Spencer, H. 1850 (1888). *Social Statics*. New York: Appleton-Century-Crofts.

Spencer, H. 1884. *The Man Versus the State with Six Essays on Government, Society, and Freedom*. New York: D. Appleton.

Stacey, J. and Throne, B. 1985. The missing feminist revolution in sociology. *Social Problems,* 32, 301–16.

Stivens, Maila. 2000. Introduction: gender politics and the reimagining of human rights in the Asia Pacific, in *Human Rights and Gender Politics: Asia-Pacific Perspectives,* edited by A. Hilsdon, V. Mackie, M. Macintyre, and M. Stivens. London: Routledge.

Straubs, D., Loch, K., Evaristo, B, Karahanna, E. and Srite, M. 2002. Toward a theory-based measurement of culture. *Journal of Global Information Management*, 10 (1), 13–23.

Stuart, K. 2000. The HIV/AIDS pandemic: human rights, societal, and development issues. *Interdisciplinary Science Reviews*, 25 (4), 307–405.

Tay, L.S. and Gibbons, J.L. 1998. Attitudes toward gender roles among adolescents in Singapore. *Cross-Cultural Research*, 32 (3), 257–78.

Tayor-Gooby, P. 1991. Welfare state regimes and welfare citizenship. *Journal of European Social Policy*, 1 (2), 93–105.

Thistle, S. 2000. The trouble with modernity: gender and the remaking of social theory. *Sociological Theory*, 18 (2), 275–88.

Thomas, D. 1990. Intrahousehold resource allocation: an inferential approach. *Journal of Human Resources*, 25 (4), 634–64.

Tocqueville, A. 1990 (1835). *Democracy in America Vol. 1*. (edited by P. Bradley), New York: Random House.

Togunde, O.R. 1999. Determinants of women's employment in urban Nigeria: the impact of sociocultural factors. *Journal of Asian and African Studies,* 34 (3), 279–97.

Turner, J.H. 1998. *The Structure of Sociological Theory.* Belmont, CA: Wadsworth Publishing.

Turner, B.S. 2001. The erosion of citizenship. *British Journal of Sociology,* 52 (2), 189–210.

Udry, R. 1995. Sociology and biology: what biology do sociologists need to know? *Social Forces*, 73 (4), 1267–75.

United Nations. 1948. *The Universal Declaration of Human Rights*. Available at: http://www.un.org/en.documents/unhr/index.shtml.

United Nations. 1995. *Platform for Action. The United Nations Fourth World Conference on Women* (Beijing, China, September 1995). Available at: http://www.un.org/womenwatch/daw/beijing/platform/plat1.htm.

United Nations. 1999. *Resolutions and Decisions adopted by the General Assembly during its Twenty-first Special Session*, 30 June to 2 July 1999, Supplement No. 2. A/S–21/7 section III, annex. United Nations, New York.

United Nations. 2000a. *UN Millennium Declaration*. Available at: http://www.un.org/millennium/declaration/ares552e.pdf.

United Nations. 2000b. *UN Millennium Development Goals*. Available at: http://www.un.org/millenniumgoals.

United Nations. 2002. *Human Rights: A Compilation of International Instruments of the United Nations*. Available at: www.ohchr.org/Documents/publications/compilation2en.pdf.

United Nations. 2009. *The Millennium Development Goals Report 2009*. Available at: www.un.org/millenniumgoals/pdf/MDG_Report_2009_EN.pdf.

United Nations Children's Fund (UNICEF). 2004. *The State of the World's Children*. Available at: www.unicef.org/sowc04/sowc04_tables.html.

United Nations Children's Fund (UNICEF). 2008. *The State of the World's Children 2008*. Available at: www.unicef.org/sowc08.

United Nations Children's Fund (UNICEF). 2009. *The State of the World's Children 2008–2009*. Available at: www.unicef.org/SOWC09/docs/SOWC09-ExecSummary-EN.pdf.

United Nations Children's Fund (UNICEF), WHO and UNFPA. 1997. *Guidelines for Monitoring the Availability and Use of Obstetric Services*. New York: UNICEF. Available at: www.unicef.org.

United Nations Development Fund for Women. 2001. *Progress of the World's Women 2000*. Available at: www.unifem.undp.org/progressww/2000.

United Nations Development Programme (UNDP). 1974. *Report of the United Nations World Population Conference*, 1974, Bucharest, 19–30 August 1974, New York: United Nations.

United Nations Development Programme (UNDP). 1990. *Human Development: Concept and Measurement of Human Development*. Available at: http://hdr.undp.org/reports/global/hdr1990.

United Nations Development Programme (UNDP).1994. *Cairo Programme of Action*. Available at: http://www.un.org/ecosocdev/geninfo/population/icpd.htm.

United Nations Development Programme (UNDP). 1995. *Human Development Report 1995*. Available at: http://hdr.undp.org/reports/global/1995.

United Nations Development Pragramme (UNDP). 2000. *Human Development Report 2000*. Available at: http://hdr.undp.org/reports/global/2000.

United Nations Development Pragramme (UNDP). 2001. *Human Development Report 2001*. Available at: http://hdr.undp.org/reports/global/2001.

United Nations Development Programme (UNDP). 2003. *Human Development Report 2003*. New York: Oxford University Press.

United Nations Development Programme (UNDP). 2004. *Human Development Report: Cultural Liberty in Today's Diverse World*. Available at: http://hdr.undp.org/reports/global/2004.

United Nations Development Programme (UNDP). 2006. *Millennium Development Goals*. Available at: www.undp.mdg.

United Nations Development Programme (UNDP). 2006. *Taking Gender Equality Seriously: Making Progress, Meeting New Challenges*. Available at: www.undp.org/women/docs/TakingGenderEqualitySeriously.pdf.

United Nations Development Programme (UNDP). 2008. *Human Development Report 2007–2008* Available at: http://hdr.undp.org/en/media/HDR_20072008_EN_complete.pdf.

United Nations Economic and Social Affairs. 2006. *World Population Prospects: The 2006 Revision*. Available at: www.un.org/esa/population/publications/wpp2006/English.pdf.

United Nations Economic and Social Commission for Asia and the Pacific (ESCAP). 1998. *Regional Prospects for Social Development: An Overview*. Bangkok: United Nations.

United Nations Fund for Population Activities (UNFPA). 2000. *Reproductive Health in Refugee Situations*. Available at: www.unfpa.org/emergencies/manual/2.htm.

United Nations Fund for Population Activities (UNFPA). 2002. *Ensuring Reproductive Health and Rights would Go a Long Way in Overcoming Poverty*. Available at: www.globalpolicy.org/socecon/develop/2002.

United Nations Fund for Population Activities (UNFPA). 2003. *The State of World Population 2003*. Available at: www.unfpa.org/swp/2003/pdf/english/swp2003_eng.pdf.

United Nations Fund for Population Activities (UNFPA). 2004a. *Women and HIV/AIDS: Confronting the Crisis*. Available at: www.unfpa.org.

United Nations Fund for Population Activities (UNFPA). 2004b. *The State of World Population 2004*. Available at: www.unfpa.org/swp/2004/pdf/english/swp2003_eng.pdf.

United Nations Fund for Population Activities (UNFPA). 2005. *The State of World Population 2005.* Available at: www.unfpa.org/upload/lib_pub_file/493_filename_en_swp05.pdf.

United Nations Fund for Population Activities (UNFPA). 2008. *The State of World Population 2008*. Available at: www.unfpd.org/swp/2008/en.

United Nations Fund for Population Activities (UNFPA). 2009. *The State of World Population 2004–2009*. Available at: www.unfpa.org.

United Nations Fund for Population Activities (UNFPA) and Population Reference Bureau (PRB). 2003. *Country Profiles for Population and Reproductive Health: Policy Developments and Indicators 2003*. Available at: www.unfpa.org/upload/lib_pub_file/200_filename_profiles2003_final.pdf.

United Nations Fund for Population Activities (UNFPA) and Population Reference Bureau (PRB). 2005. *Country Profiles for Population and Reproductive Health: Policy Developments and Indicators 2003*. Available at: www.unfpa.org/upload/lib_pub_file/200_filename_profiles2005_final.pdf.

United Nations High Commissioner for Refugees (UNHCR). 2008. *2008 Global Trends: Refugees, Asylum-Seekers, Returners, Internally Displaced and Stateless Person*s. Available at: www.unhcr.org/4a375c426.html.

United Nations International Conference on Population and Development (ICPD). 1994. *Programme of Action 1994*. Available at: www.iisd.ca/linkages/Cairo.html.

United Nations Joint Programme on HIV/AIDS (UNAIDS). 2004a. *Report on Global AIDS Epidemic*. Available at: www.unaids.org.

United Nations Joint Programme on HIV/AIDS (UNAIDS). 2004b. *A Global Overview of the AIDS Epidemic*. Available at: www.unaids.org.

United States Agency for International Development (USAID), Office of Sustainable Development.1999. *Health and Family Planning Indicators* Volume 1. Available at: http://pdf.usaid.gov/pdf_docs/PNACM806.pdf.

United States Agency for International Development (USAID). 2006. *Natural Resources and Conflict*. Available at: www.usaid.gov/our_work/cross-cutting_programs/conflict/focus-areas/natural_resources.html.

United States Census Bureau. 1993. *Money Income of Households, Families, and Persons in the United States, 1992*. Available at: http://www.census.gov.

United States Census Bureau. 2001. *Money Income in the United States: 2000*. Available at: www.census.gov/prod/2001pubs/p60–213.pdf.

Vanhanen, T. 1997. *Prospects of Democracy: A Study of 172 Countries*. London: Routledge.

Vilas, C. 1995. *Between Earthquakes and Volcanos: Market, State, and the Revolution in Central America*. New York: Monthly Review Press.

Villarreal, M. and Guerny, J. 2000. Gender and development: why do we still have problems in population programmes after all these years? *SD Dimensions*. Available at: www.unfpa.org/swp/2000/english.

Wagner, C. 1998. Slowing population growth in Ireland, Africa. *The Futurist,* 32 (8), 6–7.

Wallerstein, I. 1974. *The Modern World System: Capitalist Agriculture and Origins of the European World Economy in the Sixteenth Century*. New York: Academic Press.

Wallerstein, I. 1979. *The Capitalist World Economy*. New York: Cambridge University Press.

Wallerstein, I. 1982. The rise and future demise of the world capitalist system: concepts for comparative analysis, in *Studies on a Just World Order: Volume I: Toward a Just World Order,* edited by R. Falk, S.S. Kim, and S.H. Mendlovitz. Boulder, CO: Westview Press.

Wallerstein, I. 1984. *The Politics of the World Economy: The States, the Movements, and the Civilizations*. Cambridge, UK: Cambridge University Press.

Wallerstein, I. 1993. The present state of the debate on world inequality, in *Development and Underdevelopment: The Political Economy of Inequality*, edited by M.A. Seligson and J.T. Passe-Smith. Boulder, CO: Lynne Rienner.

Walsh, J., Mollmann, M. and Heimburger, A. 2008. Abortion and human rights: examples from Latin America. *IDS Bulletin*, 39 (3), 28–39.

Wang, G.Z. 2004. Reproductive health in the context of economic and democratic development: an analysis of developing countries. *Comparative Sociology*, 3 (2), 135–62.

Wang, G.Z. 2007. Testing the impact of gender equality on reproductive health: an analysis of developing countries. *The Social Science Journal* 44, 507–524.

Wang, G. Z. and Pillai, V.K. 2001. Women's reproductive health: a gender-sensitive human rights approach. *Acta Sociologica*, 44 (3), 231–42.

Weber, M. 1904–05. *The Protestant Ethics and the Spirit of Capitalism.* New York: Scribner's.

Weber, M. 1921. *Economy and Society* (3 volumes). Totowa, NY: Bedminster Press.

Weber, M. 1947. *The Theory of Social and Economic Organization*. Glencoe, IL: The Free Press.

Weinrobe, M. 1974. Household production and national production: an improvement of the record. *Review of Income and Wealth*, 20, 89–102.

Weiss, J.A., Ramirez, F.O. and Tracy, T. 1976. Female participation in the occupational system: a comparative institutional analysis. *Social Problems,* 23, 593–608.

Weissbrodt, D.S. 1988. Human rights: a historical perspective, in *Human Rights*, edited by P. Davis. New York: Routledge.

Weitz, S. 1977. *Sex Roles: Biological, Psychological, and Social Foundations*. New York: Oxford University Press.

Wejnert, B. 2008. Effects of global democracy on women's reproductive health 1970–2005, cross-world analysis. *Marriage and Family Review*, 44 (2/3), 154–72.

Whyte, M.K. 1978. *The Status of Women in Preindustrial Societies*. Princeton, NJ: Princeton University Press.

Wickrama, K.A.S. and Lorenz, F. 2002. Women's status, fertility decline, and women's health in developing countries: direct and indirect influence of social status on health. *Rural Sociology*, 67 (2), 255–77.

Wilkinson, R.G. 1996. *Unhealthy Societies: The Afflictions of Inequality*. London: Routledge.

Wittrock, B. 2000. Modernity: one, none, or many: European origins and modernity as a global condition. *Daedalus*, 129, 31–60.

Women's Commission for Refugee Women and Children (WCRWC). 2006. *Moving up the Food Chain: Lessens from Gender Mainstreaming at the World Food Program*. Available at: www.womenscommission.org/pdf/wfp_agdm.pdf.

Woodward, D. and Simms, A. 2006. *Growth Isn't Working: the Unbalanced Distribution of Benefits and Costs from Economic Growth*. London: New Economics Foundation.

World Bank. 2001. World Development Report 2000/2001: Attacking Poverty. Available at: http://web.worldbank.org.

World Bank. 2006. *World Development Report 2006: Equity and Development*. New York: Oxford University Press.

World Bank. 2008. *World Development Indicators*. Available at: http://publications.worldbank.org.

World Bank. 2009. *World Development Report 2009: Reshaping Economic Geography*. Available at: http://go.worldbank.org/K2CBHVB7H0.

World Health Organization (WHO). 1946. *Constitution of the World Health Organization.* Geneva: World Health Organization. Available at: www.who.int/goveranance/eb/who_constitution_en.pdf.

World Health Organization (WHO). 1997a. *Monitoring Reproductive Health: Selecting a Short List of National and Global Indicators*. Available at: www.who.int/reproductive-health/publications/hrp_97_26/monitoring_rh_national_global_indicators.pdf.

World Health Organization (WHO). 1997b. *Reproductive Health Indicators for Global Monitoring*. Available at: www.who.int/reproductive-health/publications/hrp_97_27/hrp_97_27_chapter2.en.html.

World Health Organization (WHO). 1999. *Reproductive Health Indicators for Global Monitoring: Report of an Interagency Technical Meeting 9–11, April 1997*. World Health Organization, Geneva.

World Health Organization (WHO). 2001. *Reproductive Health Indicators for Global Monitoring*. Available at: www.who.int/reproductive-health/publications/RHR_01_19/RHR_01_19_annex3p1.en.html.

World Health Organization (WHO). 2002. *The World Health Report: Reducing Risks, Promoting Healthy Life*. Geneva: World Health Organization.

World Health Organization (WHO). 2004. *World Health Report 2004: Changing History*. Available at: www.who.int/whr/2004/en.

World Health Organization (WHO). 2005. *Making Pregnancy Safer*. Available at: www.who.int/reproductive -health/mpr/attendants.html.

World Health Organization (WHO). 2006a. *World Health Report 2006: Working together for Health*. Available at: www.who.int/whr/2006/en/.

World Health Organization (WHO). 2006b. *Making a Difference in Countries: Strategic Approach to Improving Maternal and Newborn Survival and Health*. Available at: http://whqlibdoc.who.int/publications/2006/strategic_approach_eng.pdf.

World Health Organization (WHO). 2008. *Closing the Gap in a Generation: Health Equity through Action on the Social Determinants of Health*. Available at: http://whqlibdoc.who.int/publications/2008/9789241563703_eng.pdf.

World Health Organization (WHO). 2009. *World Health Statistics 2009*. Available at: www.who.int/whosis/whostat/2009/en/index.html.

World Health Organization (WHO) and United Nations Fund for Population Activities (UNFPA). 2004. *Summary Report of a WHO/UNFPA Technical Consultation 2–3 December 2003*. Available at: www.who.int/reproductive-health/publications.

World Health Organization, U.S. Agency for International Development, and the CORE Group. 2004. *Maternal and New Born Standards and Indicators Compendium*. Available at: www.coregroups.org.

World Health Organization Task Force on Research Priorities for Equity in Health and the WHO Equity Team. 2005. Priorities for research to take forward the health equity policy agenda. *Bulletin of World Health Organization*, 83 (12), 948–53.

Yamin, A.E. 1996. Defining questions: situating issues of power in the formulation of a right to health under international law. *Human Rights Quarterly*, 18, 398–438.

Yoder, J.D. 1999. *Women and Gender: Transforming Psychology*. Upper Saddle River, NJ: Prentice Hall, Inc.

Young, G., Fort, L. and Danner, M. 1994. Moving from the status of women to gender inequality: conceptualization, social indicators and an empirical application. *International Sociology*, 9 (1), 55–85.

Zhang, J. and Thomas, D.L. 1994. Modernization theory revisited: a cross-cultural study of adolescent conformity to significant others in Mainland China, Taiwan, and the USA. *Adolescence*, 29, 885–901.

Zolotas, X. 1983. *Economic Growth and Declining Social Welfare*. Athens: Bank of Greece.

Zuray, H., Khattab, H., Younis, N., El-Mouelhy, M. and Fadle, M. 1993. Concepts and measures of reproductive morbidity. *Health Transition Review*, 3 (1), 17–39.

Index

Abortion right 62, 68, 70, 71, 81, 119
Adaptation 26, 27
AGIL 27
Alienation 25
Alternative model 69, 86, 87, 88, 89
American Declaration of Independence 21
Amnesty International 65, 66, 161
Antenatal care 39, 44, 50, 54, 58, 68, 71, 76, 81
Anti-government individualism 24, 25
Arab states 5, 91, 92, 93, 94, 97, 98, 99, 119
Asia 5, 6, 7, 39, 91, 92, 93, 94, 95, 97, 98, 99, 100, 104, 105, 119

Beijing Platform for Action 59
Biomedical model (perspective) 5, 57, 107, 109, 110, 120
Birth control 7, 11
Birth rate 11, 41, 43
Buffer effect 35
Bureaucratic structure 27

Cairo Conference 1, 2, 14, 108
Causal attribution 118
Causal flows 19
Causal interpretation 69
Causal relationship 35
Cause-effect relationships 118
Chi-square 88, 89
Children immunized against measles 68, 70
Civil liberty 65, 66, 68, 70, 71, 75, 81
Civil rights movement 10
Cluster analysis 5, 91, 94, 96, 98
Confirmatory factor analysis 69, 81, 83
Contraceptive prevalence 39, 42, 43, 49, 50, 53, 54, 68, 71, 76
Convention on the Elimination of All Forms of Discrimination against Women 12, 13, 14, 16, 24
Cultural convergence 35
Cultural relativism 62

Demographic perspectives 1, 7, 11, 14
Developing countries 1, 2, 3, 5, 7, 8, 9, 11, 13, 15, 17, 22, 28, 32, 34, 36, 39, 57, 58, 66, 69, 71, 72, 73, 84, 85, 91, 92, 95, 98, 100, 103, 104, 105, 107, 108, 110, 111, 112, 113, 114, 115, 116, 119, 120
Division of labor 11, 25, 26, 31, 33, 59, 60, 104

East Asia/Pacific 5, 91, 92, 93, 94, 97, 98, 99, 119
Ecology of metropolitan regions 91
Economic development 2, 8, 14, 19, 23, 28, 31, 35, 36, 37, 38, 39, 41, 58, 64, 65, 68, 69, 81, 82, 84, 85, 91, 119, 120
Economic geography 91
Economic rights 22, 62, 63
Epidemiological transition 9, 39, 85
European Enlightenment 9, 19

Family planning 6, 8, 9, 15, 23, 34, 41, 43, 45, 46, 47, 48, 49, 51, 53, 54, 56, 103, 112, 113
Female earned income 61, 70, 72, 81
Female genital mutilation 10, 29, 41, 47, 53, 63
Female gross secondary enrollment 61, 68, 70, 72, 82
Feminist movement 10, 11
Freedom House 66, 68

French Revolution 21, 25

GDP per capita 64
Gender development index 36
Gender equality approach 1, 7, 10, 11, 15, 16, 17, 18, 33, 107, 108, 109, 110, 111, 120
Gender equity index 61, 68, 70, 72, 79
Gender inequality 30, 31, 36, 115
Genuine Progress Indicator (GPI) 64
Geography of health 91
Gini Index 64
Global Gag Rule 112
Globalization 36, 104
Goal attainment 26
Goodness of fit 69
Gross enrollment rate 72
Gross National Product (GNP) 64

Hedonic calculation 20
HIV/AIDS 2, 8, 13, 14, 24, 41, 46, 50, 53, 54, 100, 101, 103, 105
Human capital 36
Human development index (HDI) 60, 64
Human geography 91
Human rights 1, 3, 4, 8, 9, 10, 11, 12, 13, 14, 15, 16, 19, 21, 22, 23, 24, 26, 27, 28, 29, 38, 39, 41, 62, 65, 68, 71, 72, 81, 84, 85, 113, 117, 118, 119

Ideological egalitarianism 36
Infant mortality 2, 3, 41, 45, 49, 50, 51, 53, 54, 57, 64, 68, 70, 72, 79, 82, 84, 85, 93, 94, 98, 101, 102, 104, 105, 106, 108, 109, 111, 113,
Infants with low birth weight 58, 70, 72, 82, 94
Ingenuity gap 8
Internally displaced persons (people) 101, 102, 103, 104
International Conference on Population and Development (ICPD) 1, 4, 6, 13, 14, 15, 16, 29, 41, 56, 108
International Planned Parenthood Federation (IPPF) 57, 113
International women's health movement 11, 13, 15, 28

Iron cage of bureaucratic life 26

Justice as fairness 10

Latency 27
Latin America 3, 5, 37, 91, 92, 93, 94, 97, 98, 99, 107, 119
League of Nations 11
Least developed countries 3, 5, 10, 95, 97, 116
Liberalism 20
Life expectancy 9, 50, 54, 60, 64, 104, 105
Life span 6

Maternal-child care 5, 19, 35, 39, 58, 81, 82, 84, 85, 86, 87, 98, 99, 118, 119
Maternal health 2, 34, 48, 105
Maternal mortality 1, 3, 9, 30, 41, 42, 43, 48, 49, 50, 53, 54, 57, 64, 68, 70, 72, 82, 92, 93, 100, 102, 103, 104, 105, 108
Measurement model 69, 81, 82, 83
Mechanical solidarity 25
Millennium Development Goals (MDGs) 2, 14, 30, 105, 115
Multiple regression analysis 98, 99, 119

Nation-states 27
Natural rights 19, 20, 21, 24, 25, 62
Need-disposition 27
Neoclassical economic theory 36, 85
Neo-Malthusian thought 1, 7, 8, 9, 11, 28, 109, 120
Neonatal mortality 34, 41, 45, 52
Non-governmental organizations 6, 8, 103, 112, 113

Obstetric care 41, 42, 44, 50, 51, 53, 54, 58, 113
OLS model 99
Organic solidarity 25

Pattern maintenance 27
Perinatal mortality rate 41, 42, 45, 53
Political development 4, 5, 19, 37, 38, 39, 41, 58, 65, 66, 68, 71, 81, 82, 84, 118
Political freedom 66, 68, 70, 71, 75

Political rights 12, 21, 22, 23, 24, 62, 63, 65, 81
Population bomb 8, 11, 28
Population control 6, 8, 28
Population density 9
Population using adequate sanitation facilities 65, 68, 69, 70, 73
Population urbanized 65, 68, 69, 70, 74
Population with access to safe water 65, 68, 69, 70, 73
Program of Action 3, 59
Proposed model 5, 19, 21, 23, 25, 27, 29, 31, 33, 35, 37, 39, 40, 64, 66, 85, 86, 107, 119
Public health 1, 7, 9, 10, 15, 33, 39

Q-plot 69, 89

Red Cross 11
Refugee 101, 102, 103, 104
Regional variations 91, 92, 93, 94, 95, 97, 98, 99, 101, 103, 105, 108
Reproductive rights 1, 2, 3, 4, 7, 9, 11, 13, 14, 15, 16, 29, 32, 33, 62, 68, 112, 113
Role expectations 27, 36, 85

Seats in parliament 61, 68, 70, 72, 82, 83
Sex role theory 29, 109
Skilled attendant 34, 58
Social differentiation 35
Social entitlement 21, 22, 24, 62
Social rights 21, 62, 63, 68, 70, 71, 77, 81, 119
Socialization 30, 31
Sociology 27, 29, 35,
South Asia 5, 91, 92, 93, 94, 95, 97, 98, 99, 100, 104, 119
Squared multiple correlation (SMC) 81
Status-role 26
Steel-hard cage 26
Structural equation modeling (analysis) 5, 69, 87, 119
Structural model 69, 83, 86, 87, 88, 89
sub-Saharan Africa 5, 6, 34, 60, 91, 92, 93, 94, 95, 97, 98, 99, 100, 101, 102, 103, 104, 105, 119, 120
Sustainable development
Synthetic philosophy 2, 6, 14, 64

Terror scale 65, 66, 68, 70, 71, 81
Total fertility rate 41, 42, 43, 48, 49, 53
Tragedy of the commons 8

United Nations Development Programme 2, 5, 55, 60, 61, 64, 66, 67, 72, 97, 103, 114, 115
Universal Declaration of Human Rights 12, 16, 22, 62
Utilitarianism 10, 20

Women's human rights 3, 4, 11, 14, 15, 19, 22, 24, 28, 29, 38, 39, 41, 62, 71, 72, 81, 84, 118, 119
Women's reproductive health 1, 2, 3, 4, 5, 6, 7, 10, 11, 12, 13, 14, 15, 16, 18, 19, 28, 29, 30, 31, 32, 34, 35, 41, 42, 48, 50, 56, 57, 68, 72, 81, 82, 83, 84, 85, 86, 87, 88, 91, 92, 94, 95, 96, 98, 99, 100, 101, 102, 104, 105, 106, 107, 108, 109, 110, 111, 112, 113, 114, 115, 116, 118, 119, 120